Pocket Picture Guides

Cardiology
Second Edition

An Essential Slide Collection of Cardiology, based on the material in this book, is available. The collection consists of numbered 35 mm colour transparencies of each illustration in the book, and each section is accompanied by a slide index for easy reference. The material is presented in an attractive binder, which also contains a copy of the Pocket Picture Guide. The Essential Slide Collection is available from:

Mosby–Year Book Europe Limited
Lynton House
7–12 Tavistock Square
London WC1H 9LB
England

Pocket Picture Guides

Cardiology
Second Edition

Adam D. Timmis MA, MD, MRCP

Consultant Cardiologist,
London Chest and Newham
General Hospitals,
London, UK

M Wolfe

ISBN: 0 397 44686 1

Project Editor:	Zak Knowles
Design:	Pete 'Tex' Wilder
Illustrations:	Marion Tasker
	Lee Smith

Text set in Sabon and Frutiger by Tradespools, Frome
Produced by Bright Arts, Hong Kong
Printed and bound in Hong Kong, 1991
Reprinted in Hong Kong, 1993
Produced by Mandarin Offset in Hong Kong

For full details of all Mosby–Year Book Europe Limited titles,
please write to Mosby–Year Book Europe Limited, Lynton
House, 7–12 Tavistock Square, London WC1H 9LB, England.

PREFACE

The second edition of this Pocket Picture Guide to Cardiology has been substantially revised to include a new section of symptoms and signs of heart disease and also additional illustrative material to cover many of the emerging diagnostic technologies and therapeutic methods. Among the 148 new illustrations are examples of computed tomography, colour-flow Doppler echocardiography, magnetic resonance imaging, and a wide range of interventional catheterization techniques, including coronary angioplasty and balloon valvuloplasty. Also covered are the most recent recommendations for thrombolytic therapy in acute myocardial infarction, the management of cardiac arrest and the treatment of acute and chronic heart failure.

The book is a comprehensive and up-to-date manual of clinical cardiology suitable for all those who are seeking an introduction to this exciting medical specialty.

A.D.T.
London 1990

ACKNOWLEDGEMENTS

The author would like to thank the following colleagues for providing illustrative material: Dr. L. Allen, Guy's Hospital London (Fig. 237); M. Monaghan, King's College Hospital London (Figs. 70, 100, 111, 119, 129, 134); Dr. J. Reidy, Guy's Hospital London (Fig. 243); Dr. J.B. Timmis, Whittington Hospital London (Figs. 166, 242, 236); Dr. S.R. Underwood, Royal Brompton Hospital London (Fig. 246). Figs. 28, 30, 32, 163 provided courtesy of: Timmis AD. Disorders of the cardiovascular system. In: Trounce J and Rees PJ, eds. A New Short Textbook of Medicine. London: Edward Arnold, 1988: 3–85. Figs. 19, 24, 26, 66, 82, 120 provided courtesy of: Timmis AD. Essentials of Cardiology. Oxford: Blackwell Scientific Publications, 1988.

CONTENTS

THE NORMAL HEART

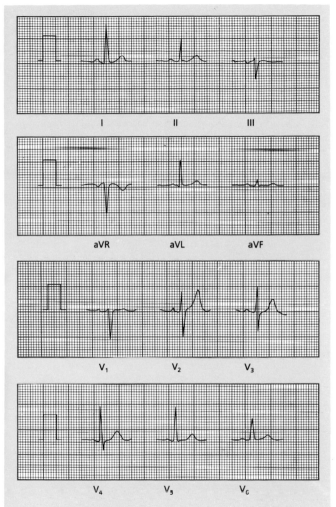

Fig.1 Electrocardiogram (ECG). This is a record of the electrical activity of the heart recorded at the skin surface. Three *bipolar* leads (I to III) and nine *unipolar* leads (aVR to V6) are usually displayed. The paper speed is 25mm per second such that each small square (1mm) represents 0.04 seconds and each large square (5mm) represents 0.20 seconds. The square wave is a calibration signal: 1cm vertical deflection – 1mV. A calibration signal should be included with every 12 lead ECG recording.

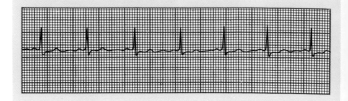

Fig.2 Sinus rhythm (lead II). The sinus node is the pacemaker of the normal heart. It depolarizes spontaneously at regular intervals which determines the heart rate. The sinus node is influenced by a variety of neurohumoral factors, particularly vagal and sympathetic activity which respectively slow and quicken the heart rate. Each sinus discharge produces atrial depolarization (P wave) followed by ventricular depolarization (QRS complex) and ventricular repolarization (T wave). This sequence of ECG deflections occurring at regular intervals is the hallmark of sinus rhythm.

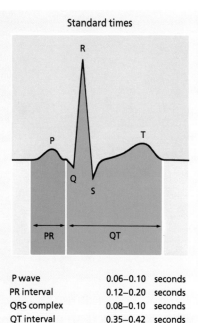

P wave	0.06–0.10	seconds
PR interval	0.12–0.20	seconds
QRS complex	0.08–0.10	seconds
QT interval	0.35–0.42	seconds

Fig.3 Note that the PR and QT intervals are both rate dependent and tend to shorten as the heart rate increases.

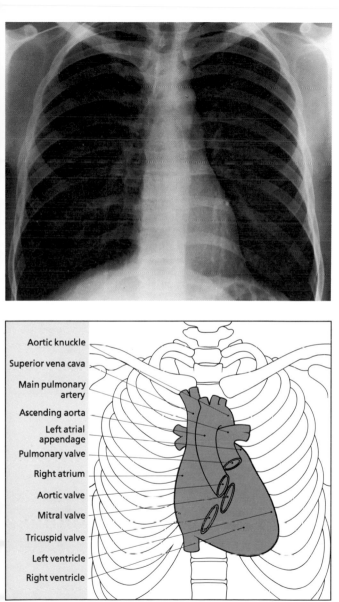

Aortic knuckle
Superior vena cava
Main pulmonary artery
Ascending aorta
Left atrial appendage
Pulmonary valve
Right atrium
Aortic valve
Mitral valve
Tricuspid valve
Left ventricle
Right ventricle

Fig.4 Chest X-ray. This is the postero-anterior projection. Note that the maximum transverse diameter of the heart should not exceed 50% the transverse diameter of the chest.

4

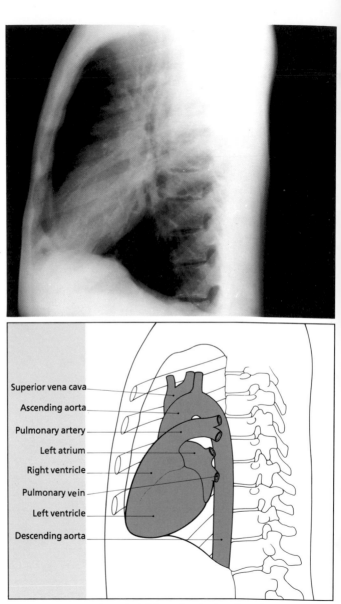

Fig.5 Chest X-ray. This is the left lateral projection. Note that the right-sided cardiac chambers lie *anterior* to the left-sided chambers.

Superior vena cava
Ascending aorta
Pulmonary artery
Left atrium
Right ventricle
Pulmonary vein
Left ventricle
Descending aorta

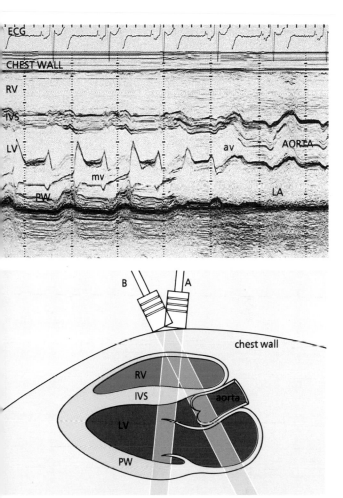

Fig.6 M-mode echocardiogram – sweep from left ventricular cavity to aortic root. The ultrasound beam provides a one-dimensional 'ice-pick' image of the heart in systole and diastole. The vertical dots are a 1 cm scale. Angulation of the beam during continuous recording permits sequential examination of the left-sided chambers and heart valves.

RV – right ventricle   av – aortic valve
LV – left ventricle   mv – mitral valve
IVS – interventricular septum
LA – left atrium
PW – posterior wall of left ventricle

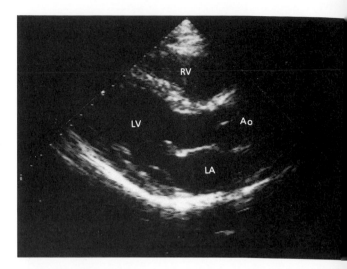

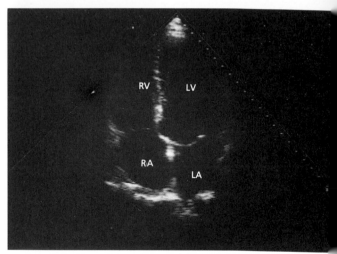

Fig.7 2-dimensional echocardiogram. (a) Parasternal long-axis view.
(b) Apical four chamber view. The images may be recorded on magnetic tap
to provide a 'real time' record of events during the cardiac cycle.
RV – right ventricle
LV – left ventricle
LA – left atrium
RA – right atrium
Ao – aorta

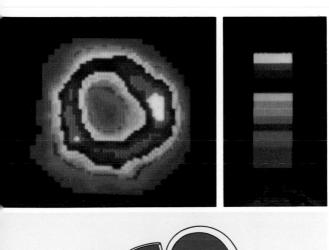

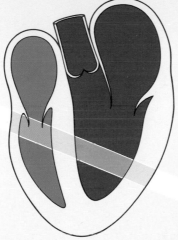

Fig.8 Myocardial perfusion scintiscan. The radionuclide thallium-201 is a potassium analogue that binds to normal cardiac myocytes. The distribution of thallium-201 in the myocardium is closely related to regional coronary perfusion. This illustration is a tomographic 'slice' through the left ventricle, imaged with a gamma camera. Colour coding shows homogeneous distribution of isotope in the myocardium (reflecting normal coronary perfusion) with negligible uptake in the LV cavity. Multiple tomographic slices at different levels may be taken to provide a record of regional perfusion throughout the myocardium. Non-homogeneous distribution of isotope is usually caused by coronary artery disease. Note that isotope uptake in the thin-walled right ventricle is normally insufficient for imaging.

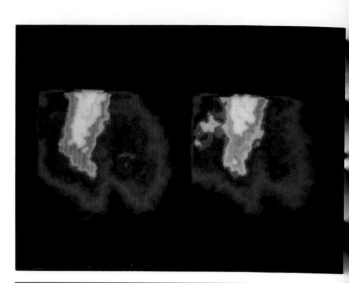

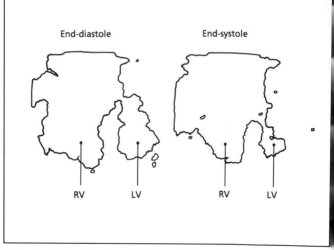

Fig.9 Equilibrium blood pool scintiscan. Left anterior oblique view. Red cells labelled with technetium-99m have been injected into a peripheral vein and allowed to equilibrate throughout the circulating blood. These colour coded images have been obtained with a gamma camera and show the peak and trough of radioactivity within the ventricular cavities after diastolic filling and systolic ejection, respectively. Analysis of wall motion obtained in this way provides a useful index of left and right ventricular function.

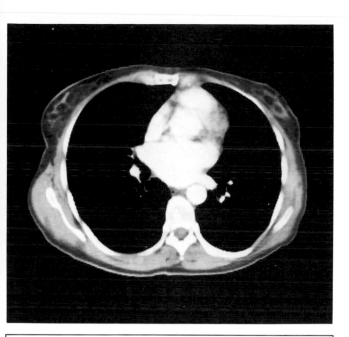

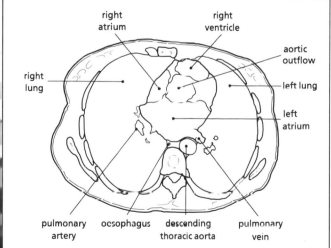

Fig.10 Computed axial tomogram. A thoracic tomogram at left atrial level is shown. The vascular spaces have been 'enhanced' by the injection of contrast solution into the bloodstream.

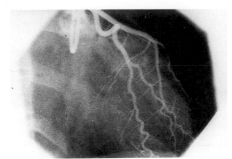

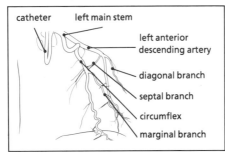

catheter   left main stem

left anterior
descending artery

diagonal branch

septal branch

circumflex

marginal branch

Fig.11 Coronary arteriograms. Right anterior oblique views. A catheter has been introduced through the right brachial artery and directed into the ascending aorta. The tip of the catheter has been positioned first in the left and then the right coronary ostium. Contrast material injected through the catheter provides X-ray images of the coronary arterial tree.

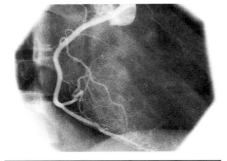

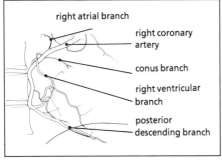

right atrial branch

right coronary
artery

conus branch

right ventricular
branch

posterior
descending branch

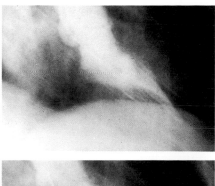

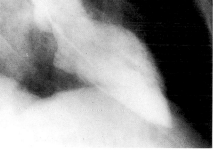

Fig.12 Left ventriculogram. Right anterior oblique views. The catheter has been passed from the ascending aorta through the aortic valve into the LV cavity. These are systolic and diastolic frames from a cine-angiogram performed during injection of contrast material.

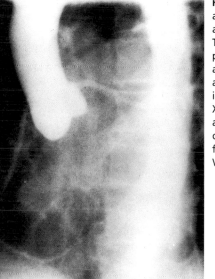

Fig.13 Aortic root angiogram. Left anterior oblique view. The catheter has been pulled back across the aortic valve into the aortic root. A contrast injection provides an X-ray image of the ascending aorta. The coronary arteries arising from the sinuses of Valsalva are clearly seen.

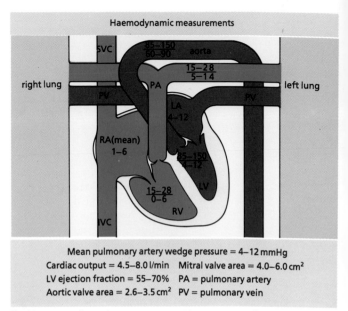

Haemodynamic measurements

SVC

$\dfrac{85-150}{60-90}$ aorta

$\dfrac{15-28}{5-14}$

right lung

PV   PA   PV   left lung

LA
4–12

RA(mean)
1–6

$\dfrac{85-150}{5-12}$

$\dfrac{15-28}{0-6}$ LV

RV

IVC

Mean pulmonary artery wedge pressure = 4–12 mmHg
Cardiac output = 4.5–8.0 l/min   Mitral valve area = 4.0–6.0 cm²
LV ejection fraction = 55–70%   PA = pulmonary artery
Aortic valve area = 2.6–3.5 cm²   PV = pulmonary vein

Fig.14 Haemodynamic measurements. These are normal pressures (mmHg) measured at rest.

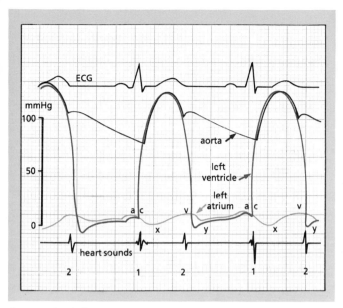

Fig.15 Left-sided pressure signals. Simultaneous recordings of the aortic, left ventricular and left atrial pressure signals are shown. At the end of diastole, following atrial contraction, the sharp rise in left ventricular pressure forces closed the mitral valve ('c' wave). As left ventricular pressure exceeds aortic pressure the aortic valve opens to allow ejection of blood. Thereafter the pressures in the left ventricle and aorta remain equal and superimposed until aortic valve closure occurs, corresponding to the dicrotic notch. Throughout diastole the decline in aortic pressure is relatively gradual as blood runs off into the peripheral circulation. Left ventricular pressure, on the other hand, falls precipitately and, as it drops below left atrial pressure, the mitral valve opens to allow ventricular filling. This checks the decline in left ventricular pressure, which rises slowly until the onset of systole leads to closure of the mitral valve and initiates another cycle.

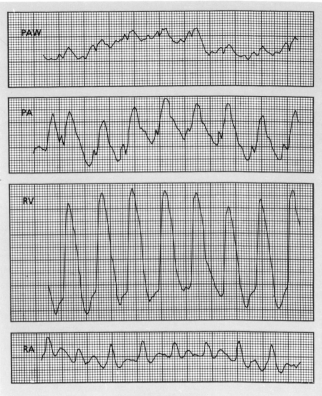

Representative values

PAWP – 9 mmHg
PA – 26/9 mmHg
RV – 26/3 mmHg
RA – 3 mmHg

Fig.16 Right-sided pressure signals. A flexible balloon-tipped catheter (*Swan Ganz catheter*) has been inserted into a central vein and guided through the right side of the heart into a branch of the pulmonary artery. Inflation of the balloon occludes the pulmonary arterial branch and the pressure recorded at the catheter tip (pulmonary artery wedge – PAW— pressure) is a measure of the left atrial pressure transmitted 'backwards' through the pulmonary capillary bed. Deflation of the balloon permits measurement of the pulmonary artery (PA) pressure. Withdrawal of the catheter through the right ventricle (RV) and right atrium (RA) provides a record of the intracardiac pressure signals.

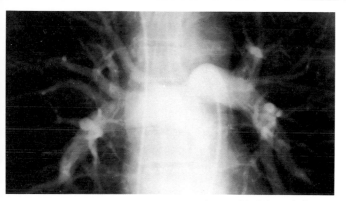

Fig.17 Pulmonary angiogram. A catheter has been guided through the right side of the heart and positioned in the main pulmonary artery. Rapid injection of contrast solution produces opacification of the arterial tree throughout both lung fields.

SYMPTOMS AND SIGNS OF HEART DISEASE

Cardiac causes of chest pain.				
Clinical syndrome	Typical pathology	Provocation of pain	Onset of pain	Character of pain
Angina	Coronary atheroma – smooth plaque	Exertion, anxiety, cold weather	Crescendo	Constricting
Unstable angina	Coronary atheroma – ruptured plaque with subocclusive thrombus	Unprovoked	Crescendo	Constricting
Variant angina	Coronary spasm	Unprovoked	Crescendo	Constricting
Myocardial infarction	Coronary atheroma ruptured plaque with occlusive thrombus	Unprovoked	Crescendo	Constricting
Pericarditis	Inflammatory pericardial disease	Coughing, deep inspiration	Abrupt	Sharp
Aortic dissection	Cystic medial necrosis	Unprovoked	Abrupt	Tearing
Pulmonary embolism	Ilio-femoral venous thrombosis with thromboembolism	Unprovoked	Abrupt	Constricting/ pleuritic

Fig.18 Cardiac causes of chest pain.

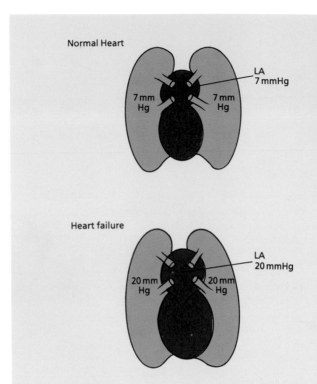

Fig.19 Dyspnoea, orthopnoea and fatigue. Exertional dyspnoea, orthopnoea and fatigue are important symptoms of heart failure. In left heart failure, the threat to cardiac output triggers reflex responses which increase left atrial pressure through central redistribution of flow and fluid retention. The increase in left atrial pressure increases left ventricular filling pressure which dilates the heart and helps maintain output by the Starling mechanism (see Fig.78). However, because there are no valves in the pulmonary veins draining into the left atrium, the rise in left atrial pressure also produces a parallel rise in pulmonary capillary pressure – predisposing to pulmonary congestion and *shortness of breath*. These symptoms are worse during *exertion* or *lying flat*, both of which produce a sharp rise in left atrial pressure. If the exertional rise in left atrial pressure fails to produce a sufficient increase in cardiac output, oxygen delivery to exercising muscle becomes inadequate and the patient experiences *fatigue*. Figs. 20-22 show the effects of exercise and altered posture on pulmonary artery wedge pressure (PAWP) and cardiac output in patients with heart failure, compared with normal individuals. PAWP is an indirect measure of left atrial pressure (see Fig.89).

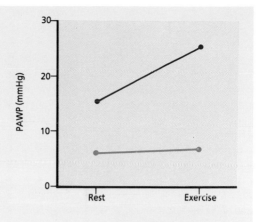

Fig.20 Dyspnoea. Exercise has little effect on PAWP in the normal individual (⟷) but provokes a sharp rise in the patient with heart failure (⟷). This may lead to pulmonary congestion which contributes to the sensation of dyspnoea, although other mechanisms also play a role, including exertional acidosis, neurogenic factors and respiratory muscle fatigue.

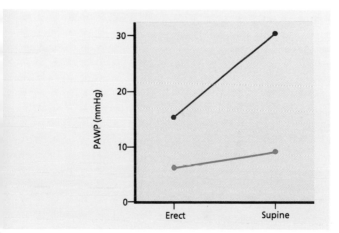

Fig.21 Orthopnoea. Gravitational pooling of blood in the upright posture ensures a relatively low PAWP, but lying flat causes it to rise sharply, particularly in patients with heart failure (⟷). This produces orthopnoea which may disturb normal sleep. In advanced cases, frank pulmonary oedema in the supine posture can cause very severe dyspnoea – *paroxysmal nocturnal dyspnoea*.

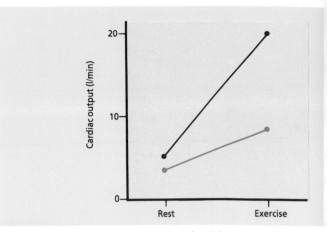

Fig.22 Fatigue. The sharp rise in PAWP (or left atrial pressure) with exertion seen in patients with heart failure may not be adequate to increase the cardiac output sufficiently to meet the oxygen requirement of exercising muscle. This produces exertional fatigue, a troublesome symptom in heart failure.

Cardiac causes of dizziness and syncope

Clinical syndrome	Aetiology	Provocation	Treatment
Postural hypotension	Baroreceptor dysfunction causing postural drop in blood pressure	Standing	None available
Vasovagal attacks	Autonomic overactivity causing bradycardia and vasodilatation with drop in blood pressure	Emotional and painful stimuli	None available
Carotid sinus syncope	Vagal overactivity caused by external pressure on carotid sinus	Tight shirt collar, shaving neck	Pacemaker
Stokes Adams attacks	Self limiting asystole or tachyarrhythmias with no effective cardiac output	None	Pacemaker and/or antiarrhythmic drugs
Valvar obstruction	Aortic stenosis, left atrial myxoma	Exercise	Surgery

Fig.23 Cardiac causes of dizziness and syncope. Cardiovascular disorders cause dizziness and syncope by transient disturbance of cerebral perfusion. Recovery usually occurs within a few minutes, unlike other common causes of unconsciousness (e.g., stroke, epilepsy, overdose) in which full recovery may take several hours.

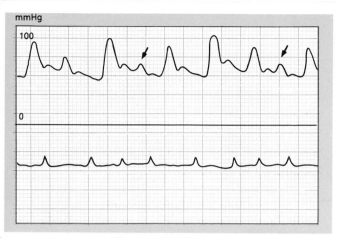

Fig.24 Pulse rate – atrial fibrillation. Simultaneous recording of the ECG and radial artery pressure signal in atrial fibrillation. The pulse rate is usually assessed by palpating the radial pulse. In atrial fibrillation, however, accurate rate assessment requires auscultation of the heart with a stethoscope because beats following very short diastolic intervals (arrowed) may not generate sufficient pressure for palpation at the wrist.

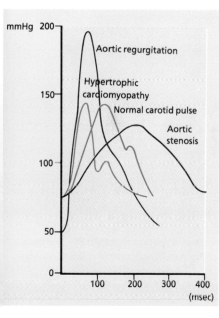

Fig.25 Pulse character. The pulse is generated by the left ventricle, and the waveform (*character*) is best assessed by palpation of the right carotid artery – the pulse closest to the heart. Abnormal waveforms are identified by the rate of the carotid upstroke.
A. Normal upstroke.
B. Rapid upstroke 'collapsing' pulse: aortic regurgitation.
C. Rapid upstroke 'jerky' pulse: hypertrophic cardiomyopathy.
D. Slow upstroke 'plateau' pulse: aortic stenosis.

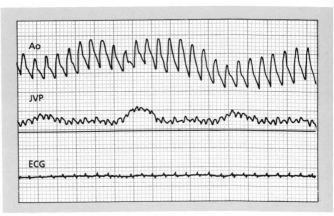

Fig.26 Paradoxical pulse and Kussmaul's sign. In this example, pericardial effusion (evidenced by the small voltage deflections on the ECG) has caused tamponade. Respiratory fluctuations in the aortic (Ao) and jugular venous pressure (JVP) signals are seen.

Paradoxical pulse – an exaggeration of the normal inspiratory decline in systolic blood pressure (>10 mmHg). Occurs in tamponade and, less commonly, in constrictive pericarditis and obstructive pulmonary disease.

Kussmaul's sign – an inspiratory rise in the JVP seen in tamponade and constrictive pericarditis. Note that in the normal individual, inspiration causes a *fall* in the JVP by reducing intrathoracic pressure.

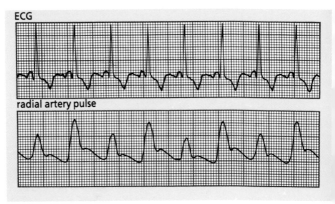

Fig.27 Pulsus alternans. Simultaneous recordings of the ECG and the radial artery pressure in a patient with heart failure. Note the alternating high and low arterial pressure deflections. Pulsus alternans is always indicative of advanced ventricular disease. The precise cause of this phenomenon is not known.

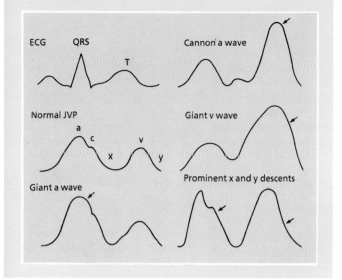

Fig.28 The jugular venous pulse. This should be assessed with the patient reclining at 45°. The JVP has a flickering character caused by the 'a' and 'v' waves.

ECG. Electrical events precede mechanical events in the cardiac cycle. Thus the P wave (atrial depolarization) and the QRS complex (ventricular depolarization) precede the 'a' and 'v' waves, respectively, of the JVP.

Normal JVP. The 'a' wave produced by atrial systole is usually the most prominent deflection. It is followed by the 'x' descent interrupted by the small 'c' wave marking tricuspid valve closure. Atrial pressure then rises again ('v' wave) as the atrium fills passively during ventricular systole. The decline in atrial pressure as the tricuspid valve opens produces the 'y' descent.

Giant 'a' wave (arrowed). This is caused by forceful atrial contraction against a stenosed tricuspid valve or a noncompliant hypertrophied right ventricle.

Giant 'v' wave (arrowed). This is an important sign of tricuspid regurgitation. The regurgitant jet produces pulsatile systolic waves in the JVP (see Fig.135).

Cannon 'a' wave (arrowed). This is caused by atrial systole against a closed tricuspid valve. It occurs when atrial and ventricular rhythms are dissociated (complete heart block, ventricular tachycardia) and marks coincident atrial and ventricular systole.

Prominent 'x' and 'y' descents (arrowed). These occur in constrictive pericarditis and give the JVP an unusually dynamic appearance (see Fig.170). In tamponade, only the 'x' descent is exaggerated.

First heart sound (S1).	
Loud S1	Mitral stenosis (mild/moderate)
Soft S1	Mitral stenosis (very severe)
Variable S1	AV dissociation (complete heart block, ventricular tachycardia)

Fig.29 First heart sound (S1). S1 coincides with mitral and tricuspid valve closure at the onset of ventricular systole. In mitral stenosis, LV filling is prolonged and the valve leaflets remain widely separated at the onset of systole. Mitral valve closure, therefore, generates unusually vigorous vibrations and S1 is loud. In very advanced mitral stenosis the valve is so rigid and immobile that S1 becomes soft again. In AV dissociation, the separation of the mitral (and tricuspid) valve leaflets at the onset of systole is variable and the intensity of S1 is correspondingly variable.

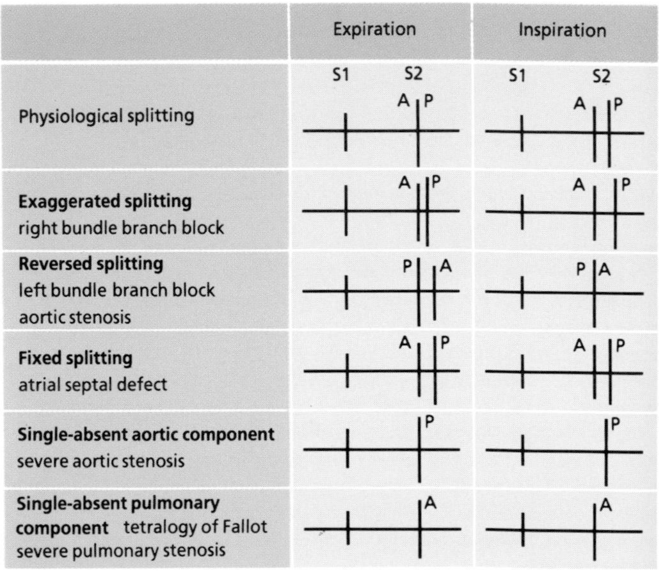

Fig.30 Second heart sound (S2). This coincides with aortic and pulmonary valve closure and marks the end of ventricular ejection. In the normal individual it is single during expiration, but during inspiration the increased venous return to the right side of the heart delays pulmonary valve closure to produce *physiological splitting* into aortic, followed by pulmonary, components. Abnormal splitting of the second heart sound is an important sign of heart disease.

	Third and fourth heart sounds (S3 and S4).	
	Normal finding	**Pathological finding**
S3	Age <35	LVF
	Pregnancy	Mitral regurgitation
		Ventricular septal defect
		Anaemia
		Fever
		Thyrotoxicosis
S4	Age >70	Hypertension
		Aortic stenosis
		Hypertrophic cardiomyopathy
		Myocardial infarction

Fig.31 Third and fourth heart sounds (S3 and S4). S3 and S4 are low frequency sounds associated with rapid ventricular filling which occurs early in diastole (S3) following mitral/tricuspid valve opening, and again late in diastole (S4) due to atrial contraction. When present, they give a characteristic *gallop* to the cardiac rhythm, best heard with the bell of the stethoscope at the cardiac apex.

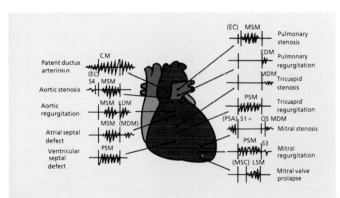

Fig.32 Heart murmurs. These are vibrations caused by turbulent flow within the heart. They are described in terms of loudness, quality, location and timing.

CM continuous murmur; MSM midsystolic murmur; PSM pansystolic murmur; LSM late systolic murmur; EDM early diastolic murmur; MDM mid-diastolic murmur; PSA presystolic accentuation; EC ejection click; MSC midsystolic click; OS opening snap; S3 third heart sound; S4 fourth heart sound.

Parentheses indicate those auscultatory findings which are not constant.

Cyanosis.			
	Pathophysiology	Physiological finding	Pathological finding
Peripheral cyanosis (skin and lips)	Desaturation of blood in vasoconstricted cutaneous circulation	Cold exposure	Heart failure
Central cyanosis (skin, lips and mucous membranes of mouth)	Desaturation of arterial blood	Never physiological	Pulmonary oedema Cyanotic congenital heart disease

Fig.33 Cyanosis. Cyanosis is a blue discolouration of the skin and mucous membranes caused by increased concentration of reduced haemoglobin in the superficial blood vessels.

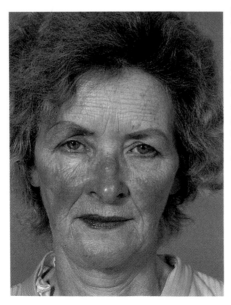

Fig.34 Mitral facies. The pronounced malar discoloration is commonly present in long standing mitral stenosis but is not specific for this condition. It is usually attributed to peripheral cyanosis associated with low cardiac output and vasoconstriction.

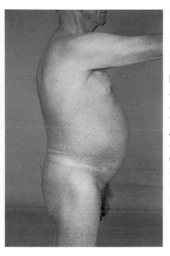

Fig.35 Ascites. Salt and water retention is a cardinal feature of heart failure and is caused by hyperaldo – steronism secondary to reninangiotensin activation. Dependent 'pitting' oedema of the ankles is an early manifestation but, as fluid overload increases, it extends to involve the legs, genitalia, trunk and abdominal viscera. In this example, effusion into the peritoneal cavity has caused ascites in a patient with constrictive pericarditis. Effusion into the pleural and pericardial spaces may also occur.

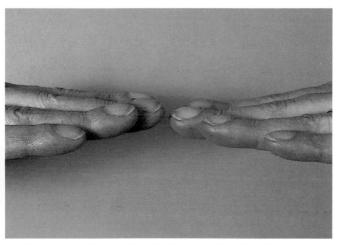

Fig.36 Clubbing. This may affect the fingers and toes. It is almost invariable in congenital cyanotic heart disease but is now an unusual feature of infective endocarditis. It may also occur in pulmonary heart disease.

CORONARY ARTERY DISEASE

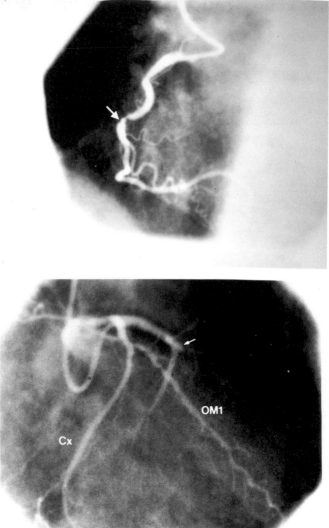

Fig.37 Coronary artery disease – the anatomical substrate. Contrast injections into the right (top) and left coronary arteries are shown. Note the tight stenosis in the right coronary artery (arrowed) and total occlusion of the left anterior descending artery (also arrowed). Irregularities are seen clearly in the first obtuse marginal (OM1) branch of the circumflex (Cx) artery.

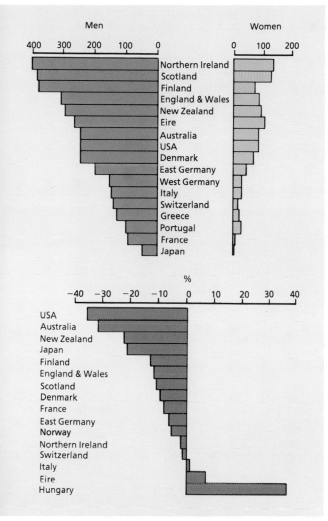

Fig.38 Mortality rates from coronary heart disease. The UK has almost the highest mortality from coronary heart disease in the world. In many countries, notably the USA and Australia, mortality has shown a sharp decline in recent years (1973-1983) but there has been little change in the UK. The reasons for this are complex but probably reflect, at least in part, attitudes to risk-factor modification which have been very positive in the USA, in contrast to the UK where this aspect of disease prevention has received much less attention.

Chronic stable angina – diagnostic strategy. Myocardial ischaemia results from an imbalance between myocardial oxygen supply and demand, and produces chest pain called angina. The history obtained from the patient provides the most useful diagnostic information. A typical history describes the pain as central in the chest, often with radiation to the arms, throat or jaw. It has a constricting quality and is provoked by stimuli which increase the oxygen demand of the heart, such as exertion or heightened emotion. The pain subsides with rest, usually after 5-10 minutes,

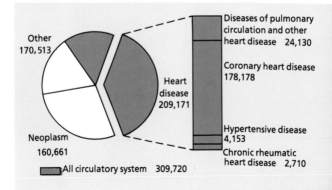

Fig.39 Causes of death in the UK in 1987. Note that circulatory disease accounts for more than half of all deaths, with coronary heart disease the major offender.

Risk factors for coronary artery disease

Potentially reversible

Tobacco smoking	Risk rises in proportion to the amount of tobacco smoked
Hypertension	Risk rises in proportion to the level of systolic and diastolic blood pressure
Hyperlipidaemia	Hypercholesterolaemia is the major risk factor, but hypertriglyceridaemia may be important in women. Elevation of low-density lipoproteins (50% cholesterol) increases the risk considerably. High-density lipoproteins (20% cholesterol), however, are protective against the disease
Obesity	The increased risk is due largely to associated hypertension, hypercholesterolaemia and diabetes
Physical inactivity	Evidence is inconclusive. Nevertheless, exercise increases high-density lipoproteins and in some individuals lowers resting blood pressure, both of which might protect against the disease
Diet	Although high-cholesterol diet, and excessive alcohol and coffee consumption, have all been associated with increased risk, the evidence is inconclusive

Irreversible

Family history	The familial incidence of coronary artery disease is largely the result of genetic predisposition to hypertension, hypercholesterolaemia and diabetes
Advanced age	Risk rises progressively with age
Male sex	Risk is low in young women, but after the menopause it increases and comes to equal that of men
Diabetes mellitus	This increases the risk in both men and women
Personality type	Although the type A personality (chronic sense of time urgency) has been associated with an increased risk compared with the more placid type B personality, the evidence remains inconclusive

Fig.40 Risk factors for coronary artery disease.

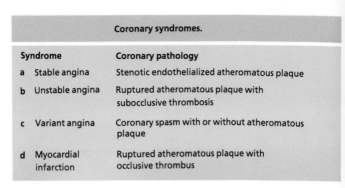

Coronary syndromes.	
Syndrome	**Coronary pathology**
a Stable angina	Stenotic endothelialized atheromatous plaque
b Unstable angina	Ruptured atheromatous plaque with subocclusive thrombosis
c Variant angina	Coronary spasm with or without atheromatous plaque
d Myocardial infarction	Ruptured atheromatous plaque with occlusive thrombus

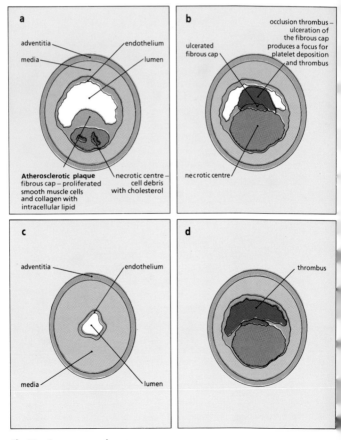

Fig.41 Coronary syndromes.

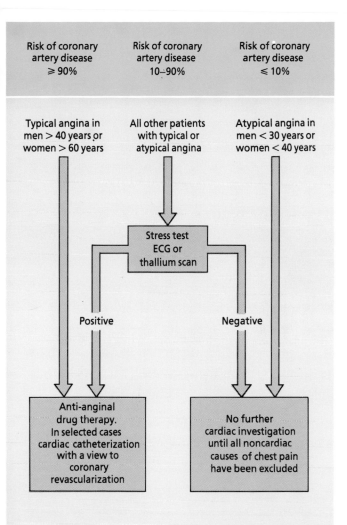

Fig.42 If the history is typical, the probability of coronary artery disease is high, exceeding 90% in men >40 years and women >60 years. If the history is atypical the probability of coronary artery disease is lower, falling below 10% in men <30 years and women <40 years. At these extremes of probability, non-invasive stress testing (ECG or thallium imaging) is of marginal diagnostic value and is not often necessary. Patients with an intermediate probability of coronary artery disease, should undergo stress testing to help confirm or refute the diagnosis of coronary artery disease.

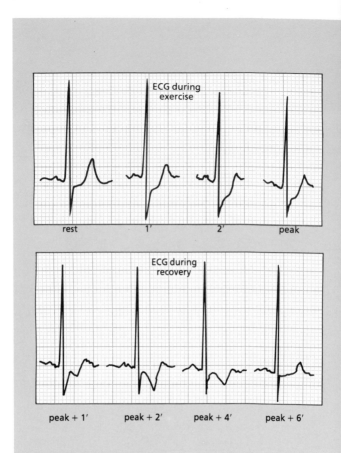

Fig.43 Exercise ECG showing lead V4 in a middle-aged man with angina exercised on a treadmill. The exercise ECG provides two different types of information in patients with suspected coronary artery disease:

1. *Diagnostic information*: exercise-induced *planar* or *downsloping* ST depression (>0.1 mV) with reversal during recovery (as shown in this example) indicates a high diagnostic probability of coronary artery disease, particularly when the history is typical. Note that false positive results are common in young women.

2. *Prognostic information*: a high risk of myocardial infarction or sudden death is indicated by ST depression very early during exercise (as shown in this example), an exertional *fall* in blood pressure or exercise-induced ventricular arrhythmias. Urgent coronary arteriography is required in these cases.

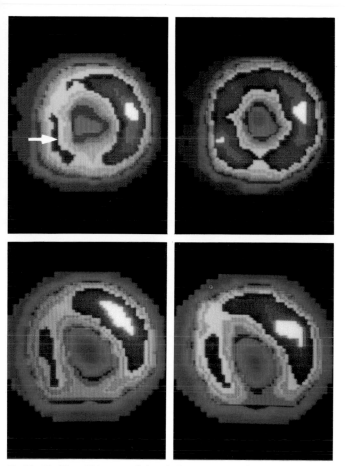

Fig.44 Thallium-201 myocardial perfusion scans at peak exercise and after three hours rest (redistribution scan).

Upper: Reversible myocardial ischaemia. The scan at peak exercise shows a clear defect in the septum (arrowed) indicating impaired perfusion. After three hours rest, however, the defect has disappeared, indicating that the ischaemia is reversible. Thus the coronary supply to this part of the myocardium is restricted but not absent. Ischaemia of this type results in angina.

Lower: Irreversible perfusion defects. The defects in the septum and inferior wall present at peak exercise show no tendency to disappear after three hours rest. This indicates irreversible myocardial damage due to previous infarction. Areas of irreversible damage do not give rise to angina since the tissue is necrosed.

| Improved myocardial oxygen delivery | | Reduced myocardial oxygen demand |

Heart rate ↓
beta blockers

Wall tension ↓
nitrates
calcium antagonists
beta-blockers

Contractility ↓
beta-blockers
(calcium antagonists)

Coronary flow
calcium antagonists
nitrates
revascularization
procedures
(bypass surgery/angioplasty)

Drug	Typical dose	echanism of action
Nitrates glyceryl trinitrate (sublingual) isosorbide mononitrate	0.4 mg PRN 20 mg b.d.	Systemic and coronary vasodilatation by direct effect on vascular smooth muscle
Beta-blockers propranolol metoprolol atenolol	40 mg tds 50 mg tds 50 mg bd	Negative chronotropic and inotropic effects by competitive blockade of cardiac beta-adrenoceptors
Calcium antagonists nifedipine diltiazem verapamil	20 mg tds 60 mg tds 40 mg tds	Systemic and coronary vasodilatation with variable negative inotropic effects by inhibition of calcium-mediated muscular contraction

Fig.45 Treatment strategies in stable angina. Correction of established risk factors is essential, particularly cigarette smoking, hypertension and hypercholesterolaemia. This must be combined with anti-anginal drug therapy. Only three groups of drugs are effective – nitrates, beta-blockers and calcium antagonists. They all improve the balance between myocardial oxygen supply and demand, but because they have different mechanisms of action their anti-anginal effects are additive when used in combination. If medical treatment fails, angioplasty or bypass surgery should be considered.

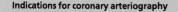

Indications for coronary arteriography

- severe angina unresponsive to medical treatment
- angina or myocardial infarction in patients under 50
- angina and a prognostically unfavourable exercise ECG
  (see Fig. 43)
- unstable angina
- angina or a positive exercise test after myocardial infarction
- cardiac arrhythmias when underlying coronary artery disease
  is suspected
- preoperatively in patients requiring valve surgery when
  advanced age (>40) or angina suggests a
  heightened probability of coronary artery disease

Fig.46 Indications for coronary arteriography. Coronary arteriography is a necessary prerequisite for revascularization by angioplasty or bypass surgery. The table shows those patients in whom coronary arteriography should be considered.

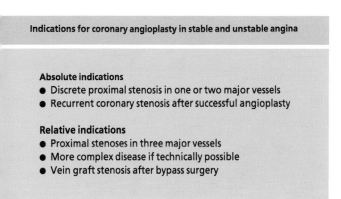

Indications for coronary angioplasty in stable and unstable angina

Absolute indications
- Discrete proximal stenosis in one or two major vessels
- Recurrent coronary stenosis after successful angioplasty

Relative indications
- Proximal stenoses in three major vessels
- More complex disease if technically possible
- Vein graft stenosis after bypass surgery

Fig.47 Indications for coronary angioplasty in stable and unstable angina.

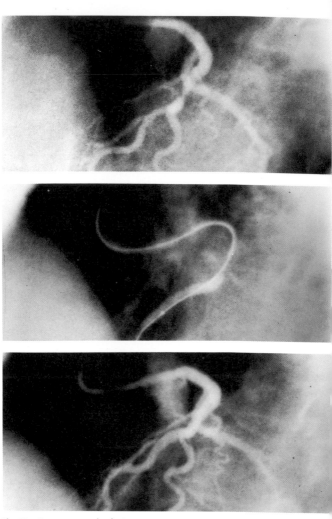

Fig.48 Coronary angioplasty.

a. Before angioplasty. A tight stenosis in the left anterior descending coronary artery is clearly demonstrated. The left coronary system is otherwise normal.

b. During angioplasty. A guide wire has been passed down the diseased vessel and a balloon catheter positioned across the lesion. The balloon is shown here inflated in order to dilate the stenosis.

c. After angioplasty. The lesion has been successfully dilated and the left anterior descending coronary artery is now widely patent.

Coronary angioplasty is less invasive and less costly than bypass surgery and offers particular advantages to the patient because hospitalization is brief and immediate return to normal activities is possible. Results are best in patients with a discrete stenosis in a single major vessel, when success can be expected in >90% of cases. As experience increases, however, excellent results are also being obtained in patients with more extensive disease. Following successful angioplasty, recurrent stenosis occurs in up to 30% of cases, requiring repeat dilatation.

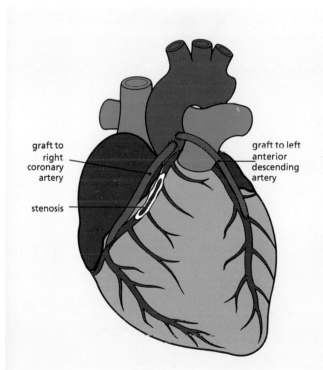

Fig.49 Coronary artery bypass grafting. Segments of saphenous vein excised from the leg of the patient have been sewn into the ascending aorta and used to bypass proximal stenoses in the left anterior descending and right coronary arteries.

It has been conclusively shown that coronary bypass surgery improves long-term prognosis in patients with left main coronary artery disease and also in patients with extensive three vessel disease, particularly when the proximal left anterior descending artery is involved. In other situations, PTCA should usually be

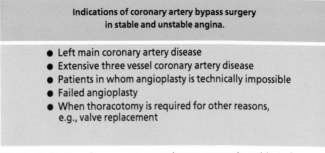

Indications of coronary artery bypass surgery in stable and unstable angina.

- Left main coronary artery disease
- Extensive three vessel coronary artery disease
- Patients in whom angioplasty is technically impossible
- Failed angioplasty
- When thoracotomy is required for other reasons, e.g., valve replacement

Fig.50 Indications for coronary artery bypass surgery in stable and unstable angina.

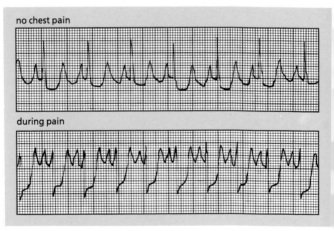

Fig.51 Unstable angina. This is caused by rupture of the atheromatous plaque with subocclusive coronary thrombosis. Profound myocardial ischaemia results in prolonged episodes of unprovoked angina, often associated with ST segment depression on the resting ECG. The ST changes reverse as chest pain subsides. Stress testing is contraindicated and unnecessary in patients with unstable angina. The diagnosis is usually clear on clinical grounds and is supported by typical ECG changes during episodes of chest pain.

considered as the potential first option, with surgery in reserve for cases in which PTCA fails or is technically impossible. Unstable angina has been called pre-infarction angina because up to 30% of patients progress to myocardial infarction within three months of presentation. Both heparin and aspirin (independently and in combination) have been shown to prevent progression to thrombotic coronary occlusion and myocardial infarction, presumably reflecting their antithrombotic properties. Whether thrombolytic drugs such as streptokinase are also useful in unstable angina remains uncertain.

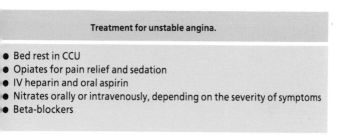

Treatment for unstable angina.

- Bed rest in CCU
- Opiates for pain relief and sedation
- IV heparin and oral aspirin
- Nitrates orally or intravenously, depending on the severity of symptoms
- Beta-blockers

Fig.52 Treatment of unstable angina.

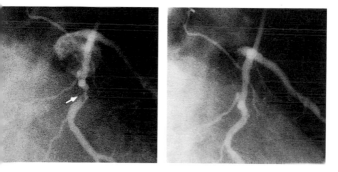

Fig.53 Revascularization in unstable angina. Revascularization by angioplasty or bypass surgery must be considered in all patients with unstable angina, particularly those who are young (<50 years) or who fail to respond to medical treatment. In this example the subocclusive coronary thrombus responsible for the unstable presentation is clearly visible (arrowed) as a filling defect in the circumflex coronary artery. Following angioplasty (right panel), the artery is widely patent enabling the patient to return to a normal life.

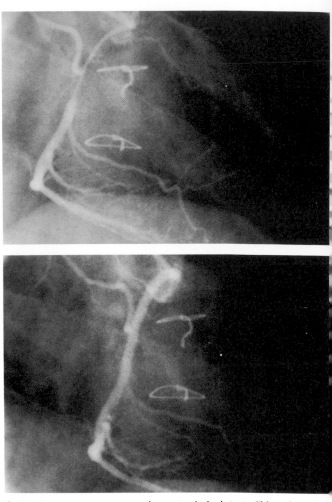

Fig.54 Coronary artery spasm – the anatomical substrate. This patient who had previously undergone mitral valve surgery was complaining of intermittent chest pain occurring at rest. Coronary arteriography demonstrated severe spasm of the right coronary artery.
Top: A long segment of the proximal right coronary artery is severely narrowed.
Bottom: Intracoronary glyceryl trinitrate corrects the abnormality and reveals a normal right coronary artery. The response to glyceryl trinitrate confirms that the narrowing was caused by spasm.

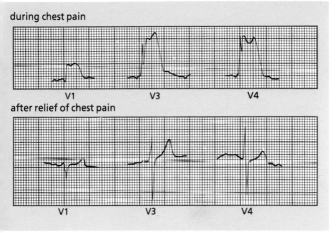

during chest pain

V1   V3   V4

after relief of chest pain

V1   V3   V4

Fig.55 Variant angina. A small group of patients exhibit reversible ST segment elevation during chest pain. This type of unstable angina is caused by episodic coronary arterial spasm often at the site of an atheromatous plaque. In about 30% of cases, however, there is no underlying atheromatous disease. Calcium antagonists prevent spasm and are the treatment of choice. Nitrates are also beneficial but beta-blockers should be avoided

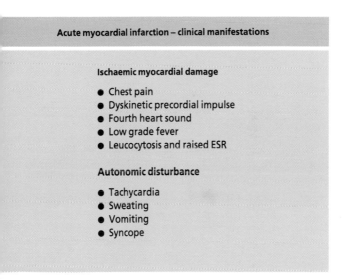

Acute myocardial infarction – clinical manifestations

Ischaemic myocardial damage

- Chest pain
- Dyskinetic precordial impulse
- Fourth heart sound
- Low grade fever
- Leucocytosis and raised ESR

Autonomic disturbance

- Tachycardia
- Sweating
- Vomiting
- Syncope

Fig.56 Acute myocardial infarction – clinical manifestations.

Diagnosis of acute myocardial infarction

The diagnosis of acute myocardial infarction can usually be made with reasonable confidence on the basis of the presenting symptoms and signs. Confirmation of the diagnosis is made by characteristic ECG and serum enzyme changes. In difficult cases non-invasive imaging techniques can provide useful additional information.

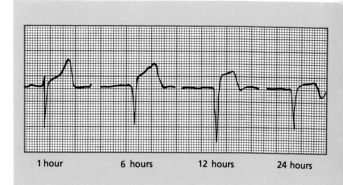

Fig.57 Evolution of ECG changes in acute myocardial infarction. The lead is V_2 in a 60 year old man. Elevation of the ST segment over the area of the infarct occurs during the first hour of chest pain. A Q wave develops during the subsequent 24 hours and usually persists indefinitely. Within a day of the attack the ST segment usually returns to the isoelectric line and T wave inversion may occur.

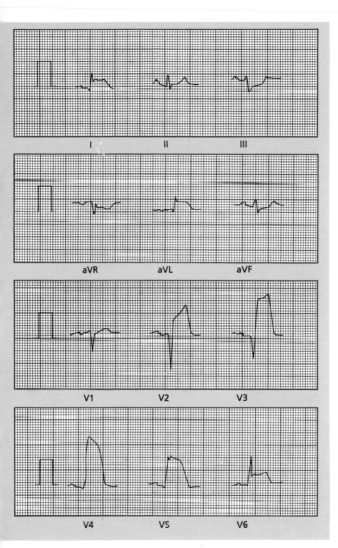

Fig.58 Acute myocardial infarction. ECG recording six hours after the onset of chest pain. Marked ST segment elevation in leads V_2 to V_6 is associated with early development of Q waves in leads V_2 and V_3. Changes in leads I and aVL indicate damage to the lateral wall. Note 'reciprocal' ST segment depression in leads III and aVF. This pattern usually reflects proximal occlusion of the left anterior descending coronary artery.

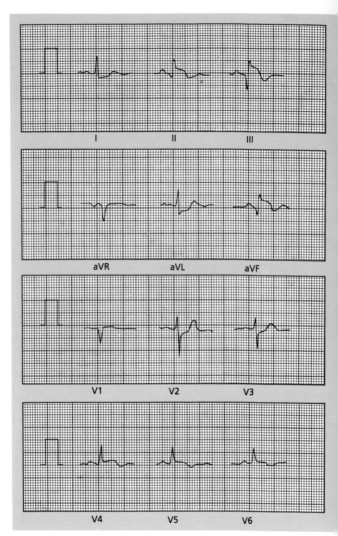

Fig.59 Acute inferior myocardial infarction. ECG recording six hours after the onset of chest pain. Typical changes are seen in leads II, III and aVF. ST segment elevation in leads V_4 to V_6 indicates lateral extension of the infarct. Note 'reciprocal' ST segment depression in leads I and aVL. This pattern usually reflects occlusion of the right coronary artery.

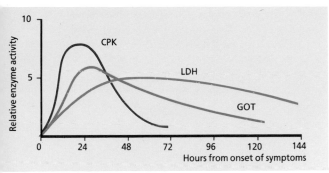

Fig.60 Time activity curves for enzymes released from the infarcted myocardium. Serum enzyme activity is expressed as multiples of the upper reference limit.

1. Creatine phosphokinase (CPK). This is the most useful enzyme clinically. Skeletal muscle is also rich in CPK and false positive results are sometimes found in patients who have received intramuscular injections.

2. Glutamic oxaloacetic transaminase (GOT). The diagnostic value of this enzyme is limited by its lack of specificity. Disease of liver, kidney, brain and lung may all give false positive results.

3. Lactic dehydrogenase (LDH). Peak levels of this enzyme occur late after infarction. Red blood cells also contain LDH and any cause of haemolysis may produce false positive results.

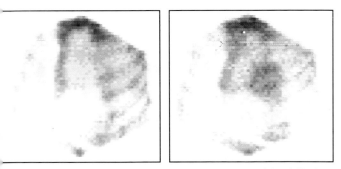

Fig.61 Hot-spot myocardial imaging. This is occasionally useful in difficult cases. Technetium-99m pyrophosphate is selectively taken up by acutely infarcted myocardium and may be imaged with a gamma camera.
Left: Normal scan. Note that isotope is taken up by normal bone and the ribs are clearly visible.
Right: Abnormal scan. Isotope has become concentrated in a large anterior myocardial infarct revealed as a dense shadow in the left side of the chest.

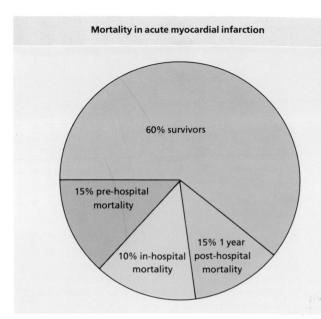

Fig.62 Mortality in myocardial infarction. These figures are approximate only, but indicate that nearly half of all patients with acute myocardial infarction die during or within one year of the attack. Most deaths occur before hospital admission and are the result of ventricular fibrillation. In hospital, however, arrhythmias can be treated, and the usual cause of death is left ventricular failure due to extensive infarction. Infarct size is also the major determinant of death in the year following hospital discharge. Thus treatment directed at limiting infarct size (particularly thrombolytic therapy) can substantially reduce mortality from myocardial infarction.

Treatment of myocardial infarction.

1. Bed rest and ECG monitoring
2. Pain relief and sedation – opiates
3. Measures to limit infarct size and reduce mortality:
   - aspirin 150 mg
   - thrombolytic therapy (see Fig. 64)
   - IV beta-blockers – atenolol 5 mg or metoprolol 5 mg
4. Anticoagulation – heparin 1000 IU/hour, starting after thrombolytic therapy
5. Treatment of complications – arrhythmias, heart failure, pericarditis

Fig.63 Treatment of myocardial infarction.

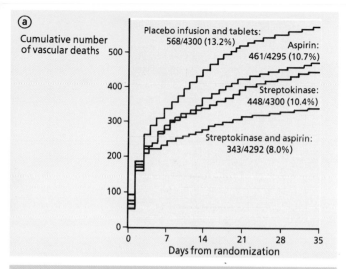

(a) Cumulative number of vascular deaths

Placebo infusion and tablets: 568/4300 (13.2%)

Aspirin: 461/4295 (10.7%)

Streptokinase: 448/4300 (10.4%)

Streptokinase and aspirin: 343/4292 (8.0%)

Days from randomization

(b) Thrombolytic drugs in acute myocardial infarction

Drug	Administration	Half-Life (minutes)	Cost per treatment (£)	Advantages	Disadvantages
Streptokinase (1.5×10^6 units)	IV Infusion	18	96	Cheap	Allergenic
Anistreplase (30 units)	IV bolus	100	495	Bolus administration	Allergenic
Alteplase (100 mg)	IV infusion	5	960	Not allergenic	Expensive

Fig.64a ISIS 2 – randomized study of streptokinase and aspirin versus placebo in acute myocardial infarction. Treatment was given within 24 hours of the onset of chest pain. More than 17,000 patients were randomized in this study which showed >20% mortality reduction at five weeks for patients who received either streptokinase or aspirin as monotherapy. The beneficial effects of these drugs were additive, and patients randomized to receive both agents showed >40% mortality reduction. A previous study from the ISIS group showed that IV beta-blocker therapy with atenolol reduces infarct mortality by about 15%. Thus current recommendations are for patients with acute myocardial infarction to receive early treatment with aspirin 160 mg, IV streptokinase (1.5 million units over one hour) and IV atenolol 5 mg. From Lancet (1988) *ii*, 349–361. **Fig.64b** Thrombolytic drugs in acute myocardial infarction.

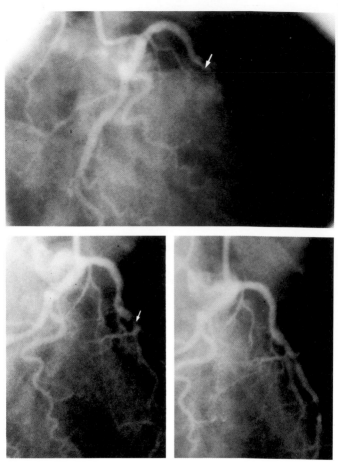

Fig.65 Thrombolytic therapy in acute myocardial infarction

A. Before streptokinase. The left anterior descending coronary artery has recently occluded (arrowed), threatening the anterior wall of the left ventricle.

B. After streptokinase. The thrombus has lysed and the artery is now patent, restoring flow to the anterior wall of the ventricle. However, there is a severe residual stenosis (arrowed).

C. After coronary angioplasty. Strategies to prevent coronary reocclusion after thrombolytic therapy may involve anticoagulant therapy or revascularization. In this case balloon dilatation of the residual stenosis was successful and the artery is now widely patent.

In acute myocardial infarction, thrombosis is the final event leading to coronary occlusion. Thrombolytic therapy lyses the thrombus and permits coronary reperfusion. If given early enough (within 24 hours of the onset of chest pain) thrombolytic therapy can salvage myocardium at risk of necrosis and reduce eventual infarct size. This lowers hospital mortality by up to 50%. Streptokinase is the most widely used drug but it depletes systemic coagulation factors and may predispose to haemorrhage, a problem not entirely avoided by the newer 'clot-specific' drugs alteplase and anistreplase. However, these newer drugs have important advantages in terms of their mode of administration (anistreplase) and their allergenic properties (alteplase).

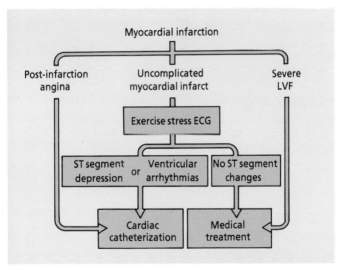

Fig.66 Management strategy after recovery from acute myocardial infarction. There is a significant risk of reinfarction and sudden death in the first year following myocardial infarction (see Fig.62). Stopping cigarette smoking and beta-blocker therapy have both been shown to reduce that risk. Residual myocardial ischaemia may have an adverse prognostic effect and for this reason exercise testing is recommended before hospital discharge. Patients with exercise-induced ischaemia (ST depression or ventricular arrhythmias) require cardiac catheterization with a view to early angioplasty or bypass surgery.

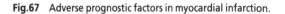

Adverse prognostic factors in myocardial infarction

1. Advanced age
2. Anterior transmural infarction
3. Left bundle branch block
4. Heart failure
5. Systolic hypotension
6. Complex ventricular arrhythmias occuring late after myocardial infarction
7. History of previous myocardial infarction

Fig.67 Adverse prognostic factors in myocardial infarction.

Complications of myocardial infarction

1. Cardiac arrhythmias
2. Heart failure
3. Pericarditis – acute
               – chronic (Dressler's syndrome)
4. Myocardial rupture – papillary muscle (mitral regurgitation)
               – interventricular septum (VSD)
               – free wall of ventricle (tamponade)
5. Thromboembolism
6. Ventricular aneurysm

Fig.68 Complications of myocardial infarction.

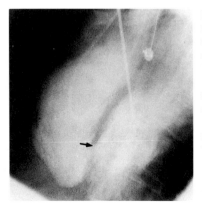

Fig.69 Myocardial rupture – ventricular septal defect. This may complicate anterior or inferior infarction. The left ventriculogram shows prompt opacification of the right ventricle due to shunting of contrast through the VSD (arrowed). Treatment is by urgent surgical repair of the defect.

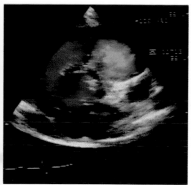

Fig.70 Myocardial rupture – ventricular septal defect. Doppler echocardiography provides a convenient non-invasive means of evaluating the direction and velocity of flow within the heart and great vessels. In this colour flow study a large jet (coloured red) is seen flowing across an apically-located VSD.

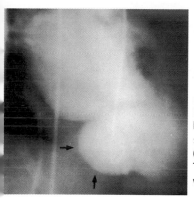

Fig.71 Myocardial rupture – papillary muscle. This is a complication of inferior infarction. The left ventriculogram shows dense opacification of the left atrium (LA) due to regurgitation through the incompetent mitral valve. The bulging dyskinetic inferior segment of the left ventricle (arrowed) is clearly visible. Treatment is by urgent mitral valve replacement.

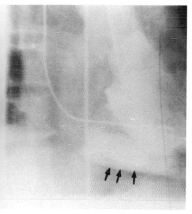

Fig.72 Myocardial rupture – free wall. Rupture of the free wall of the left ventricle usually causes rapidly fatal tamponade. In this case, however, a false aneurysm has formed in the pericardial sac protecting against tamponade. The left ventriculogram shows extravasation of contrast into the false aneurysm on the inferior surface of the heart. Treatment is by urgent surgical repair of the ruptured ventricle.

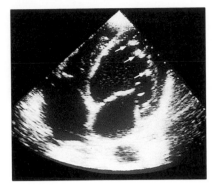

Fig.73 Mural thrombosis complicating myocardial infarction. The echocardiogram shows thrombus (arrowed) adherent to the apical and lateral walls of the left ventricle.

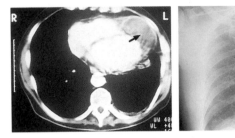

Fig.74a LV aneurysm complicating anterior myocardial infarction. This contrast-enhanced computer tomogram shows a large apical aneurysm (arrowed). It is filled with organized thrombus which has prevented penetration of contrast, such that the aneurysm appears black. LV aneurysms require no specific treatment unless they give rise to thromoembolic disease, left ventricular failure or arrythmias, in which case surgical excision may be necessary.

Fig.74b LV aneurysm. Calcification in the wall of the aneurysm may be visible on the chest X-ray several years after the acute infarct.

HEART FAILURE

Definition of heart failure

Heart failure is a syndrome in which a cardiac disorder prohibits the delivery of sufficient output to meet the perfusion requirements of metabolizing tissues

Fig.75 This definition is not all-embracing, but it serves to emphasize that the role of the normal heart is to drive the circulation. Any disturbance of cardiac function that undermines this role may result in heart failure.

Causes of heart failure				
Ventricular pathophysiology	**Clinical examples**	**Ventricle predominantly affected**		
		Left (LVF)	Right (RVF)	Both (CCF)
1. Contractile impairment	Coronary disease Cardiomyopathy Myocarditis	▇		▇ ▇
2. Pressure loading	Hypertension Aortic stenosis Coarctation Pulmonary vascular disease Pulmonary stenosis	▇ ▇ ▇	▢ ▢	
3. Volume loading	Aortic regurgitation Mitral regurgitation ASD/VSD Pulmonary regurgitation Tricuspid regurgitation	▇ ▇	▢ ▢ ▢	
4. Restricted filling	Constrictive pericarditis Tamponade Amyloidosis Mitral stenosis Tricuspid stenosis	▇	▢ ▢ ▢	▇
5. Arrhythmia	Severe bradycardia Severe tachycardia			▇ ▇

Fig.76 Causes of heart failure. Note that the separation of heart failure into LVF and RVF is to some extent artificial, since failure of one ventricle (particularly the left) leads inexorably to failure of both – resulting in congestive cardiac failure (CCF).

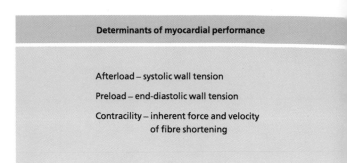

Determinants of myocardial performance

Afterload – systolic wall tension

Preload – end-diastolic wall tension

Contracility – inherent force and velocity
of fibre shortening

Fig.77 Preload, afterload and contractility are all terms derived from laboratory studies on isolated muscle. These variables are not amenable to direct measurement in the intact heart. In clinical practice the preload and afterload acting on the left ventricle are usually equated with left ventricular end-diastolic pressure and blood pressure respectively (the variables most amenable to influence by therapy), even though these pressure measurements fail to embrace the contribution that ventricular cavity dimensions make to wall tension. Contractility cannot easily be measured and is usually used qualitatively to describe the inherent force and velocity of ventricular contraction independent of loading conditions.

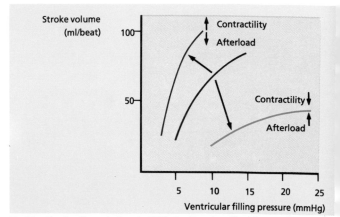

Fig.78 The Starling relation. In 1918, Starling described the curvilinear relation between preload and cardiac output. Changes in preload (or ventricular end-diastolic pressure) cause changes in output in the same direction. Later it was shown that changes in contractility and afterload influence output independently of preload, allowing a 'family' of Starling curves to be drawn. At a given preload, cardiac output changes directly with contractility and inversely with afterload.

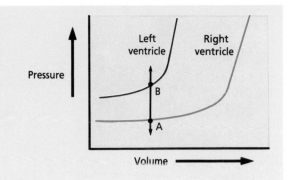

Fig.79 Ventricular pressure-volume curves. The pressure-volume relation defines the compliance characteristics of the ventricles. Note the RV curve lies below the LV curve. Thus the pressure A required to fill the thin-walled RV in diastole is appreciably lower than the pressure B required to fill the thick-walled LV to the same volume. Thus, RV diastolic pressure is lower than LV diastolic pressure.

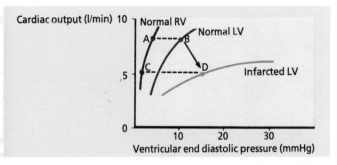

Fig.80 Disordered ventricular function in heart failure. In the normal heart RV diastolic pressure is always lower than LV diastolic pressure, but the output of the two ventricles must be the same. Thus the RV curve lies to the left of the LV curve and the ventricles operate on the same horizontal line (A-B). Myocardial infarction impairs LV contractility and the LV curve shifts down and to the right (see Fig.78). Cardiac output decreases and the ventricles must now operate on the horizontal line C-D. This involves little change in RV diastolic pressure while LV diastolic pressure increases considerably. Thus, in heart failure the discrepancy between diastolic pressures in the RV and LV is variable, depending on the relative degrees to which the function curves are depressed. Measurements of RV diastolic pressure (or central venous pressure), therefore, provide no useful information concerning LV diastolic pressure.

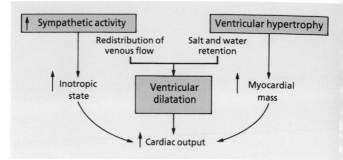

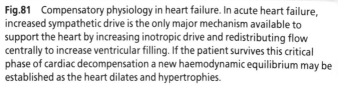

Fig.81 Compensatory physiology in heart failure. In acute heart failure, increased sympathetic drive is the only major mechanism available to support the heart by increasing inotropic drive and redistributing flow centrally to increase ventricular filling. If the patient survives this critical phase of cardiac decompensation a new haemodynamic equilibrium may be established as the heart dilates and hypertrophies.

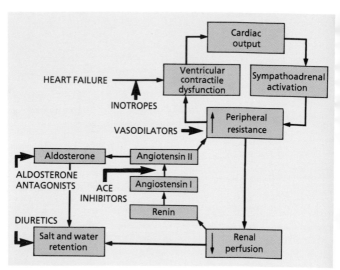

Fig.82 Neurohormonal activation in heart failure. Stimulation of the sympathoadrenal and renin-angiotensin systems helps maintain cardiac output and blood pressure. However, in the long-term this may be detrimental by the establishment of vicious cycles of falling cardiac output, increasing peripheral resistance and fluid retention. The effects of treatment are shown. Note that only angiotensin converting enzyme (ACE) inhibitors and vasodilators have the potential to break these vicious cycles.

Symptoms and signs of heart failure		
	Symptoms	Signs
Reduced cardiac output (peripheral hyperfusion)	fatigue	Cool skin Oliguria
Increased venous pressure (systemic and pulmonary congestion)	Exertional dyspnoea Orthopnoea	Cardiac enlargement Basal lung crackles Distended jugular veins Dependent oedema
Sympatho-adrenal activation	Anxiety	Tachycardia Sweating Peripheral cyanosis
Other findings		Third heart sound Pulsus alternans

Fig.83 Symptoms and signs of heart failure.

Investigation of heart failure

Chest X-ray

This provides a useful guide to the severity of pulmonary congestion in LVF. In mild cases, pulmonary venous dilatation – most marked in the upper lobes – is often the only lung–field abnormality. As failure worsens, cardiac enlargement becomes marked and, with rising pulmonary venous pressure, interstitial and finally alveolar oedema develop.

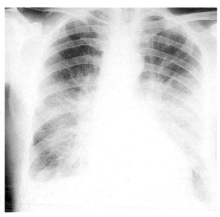

Fig.84 Chest X-ray in acute LVF. This patient has severe pulmonary oedema caused by acute myocardial infarction. The heart has not yet had time to enlarge but there is prominent alveolar pulmonary oedema in a perihilar distribution giving a typical 'bat's wing' appearance. Note the bilateral pleural effusions.

58

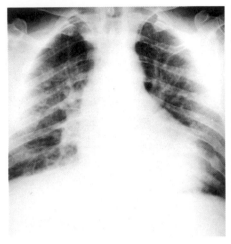

Fig.85 Chest X-ray in chronic LVF. The chest X-ray provides a useful guide to the severity of pulmonary congestion in LVF. In this example the heart is considerably enlarged and the increase in left atrial pressure (see Fig.19) has caused dilatation of the upper lobe pulmonary veins and interstitial pulmonary oedema.

Echocardiogram

This is the most useful diagnostic investigation in the patient with heart failure. It permits direct measurement of the dimensions of all the cardiac chambers and an assessment of the contractile function of the left and right ventricles. Ventricular wall thickness can also be measured. Equally important the heart valves and the subvalvar apparatus can be imaged. This technique is the most sensitive means available for detecting pericardial effusion. Thus the echocardiogram is potentially diagnostic of many of the common causes of heart failure. Four chamber dilatation and biventricular contractile failure indicates congestive cardiomyopathy. Regional wall motion abnormalities are found in ischaemic disease. Structural and dynamic valvular abnormalities with associated cavity dilatation or hypertrophy (depending on the specific lesion) permits eval-

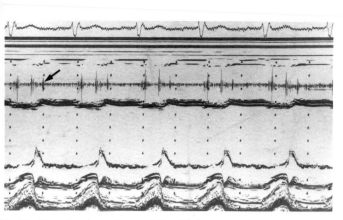

Fig.86 M-mode echocardiogram in heart failure caused by severe coronary artery disease. The heart has become stretched and dilated. Systolic function is severely impaired as reflected by the diminished excursion of the septum and, to a lesser extent, the posterior wall. The phonocardiogram (recorded simultaneously) shows normal first and second heart sounds and also S3 – a third heart sound (arrowed). S3 is a normal finding in adolescence and during pregnancy, but in most other contexts it is almost pathognomonic of heart failure.

uation of the extent and severity of valvular involvement in rheumatic, degenerative, infective and congenital disease. Pericardial effusion is readily detected in patients with tamponade.

Radionuclide imaging

This provides an alternative 'noninvasive' means of evaluating ventricular cavity dimensions and contractile function. Technetium-99m labelled red cells introduced into the circulation may be imaged with a gamma camera. The waxing and waning of scintillation counts within the ventricles during diastole and systole permits construction of a dynamic nuclear image (ventriculogram) and enables calculation of ejection fraction. Because isotope decay takes several hours, the technique is of particular value for monitoring serial responses to therapy.

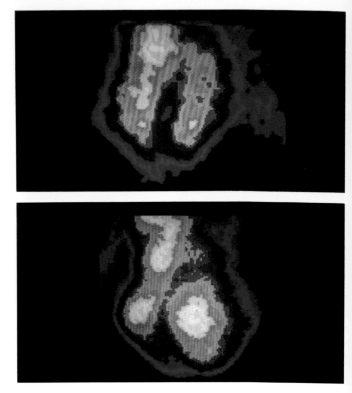

Fig.87 Radionuclide blood pool images in severe congestive heart failure. Systolic (upper) and diastolic (lower) frames are shown. In these 'colour-coded' images the greater the gamma emission the lighter the colour. The dilated ventricular cavities, therefore, are represented by the paler areas.

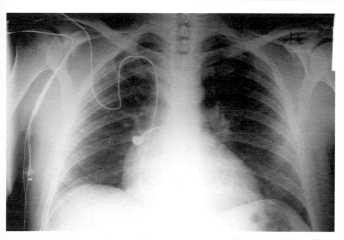

Fig.88 Right heart catheterization. A Swan-Ganz catheter is positioned in a branch of the right pulmonary artery. The catheter has a terminal balloon which, in this example, has been inflated with contrast material to improve visualization. The inflated balloon wedges in the pulmonary branch artery and occludes it; thus the tip of the catheter records the PAWP – the pressure in the pulmonary capillary system transmitted backwards from the left atrium. The PAWP is therefore a useful indirect measure of left atrial and left ventricular diastolic pressures. In LVF the PAWP is elevated but in hypovolaemic states it is low. Diagnosis and treatment of these conditions may be facilitated by monitoring the PAWP in the CCU with a Swan-Ganz catheter.

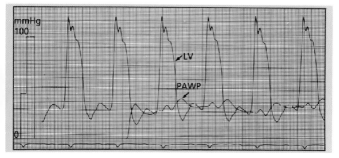

Fig.89 Simultaneous recordings of the LV pressure and PAWP. In diastole, when the mitral valve is open, the pressures are almost identical. Thus PAWP may be used as a convenient indirect measure of LV diastolic (or left atrial) pressure. In this example, the patient had severe LVF and the PAWP and LV diastolic pressures are therefore considerably elevated.

Treatment of acute left ventricular failure	
1. General measures	Sedate with morphine
	Nurse in head-up position
2. Correct aggravating factors	Arrythmias, anaemia, hypertension
3. Correct hypoxaemia	Oxygen therapy
	Mechanical ventilation if necessary
4. Specific therapy	Drugs – diuretics, vasodilators, inotropes
	Mechanical support – intra-aortic balloon pump
	Surgery – replacement of diseased valve – closure of septal defects

Fig.90 Treatment of acute LVF.

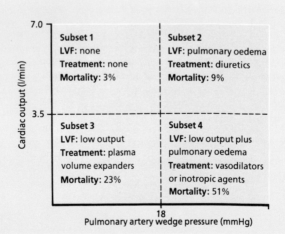

Fig.91 Treatment of acute LVF: haemodynamic subsets. A Swan-Ganz catheter with a thermodilution device permits measurement of PAWP (an indirect measure of LV diastolic pressure) and cardiac output. Pulmonary oedema usually occurs as the PAWP rises above 18 mmHg, while peripheral hypoperfusion develops as output drops below 3.5 l/min. In acute LVF, pulmonary oedema and peripheral hypoperfusion may occur independently or together and these critical values provide the basis for subset classification which may be used to guide treatment and assess prognosis.

Drugs used in acute left ventricular failure			
Drug	**Action**	**Physiology**	**Therapeutic effect**
Diuretics Frusemide (40–80 mg)	Diuresis	↓ Preload	Corrects pulmonary oedema
Vasodilators Morphine (5–10 mg)	Venodilation	↓ Preload	Corrects pulmonary oedema
Glyceryl trinitrate (10–150 μg/min)	Venodilation	↓ Preload	Corrects pulmonary oedema
Nitroprusside (25–150 μg/min)	Veno- and arteriolar dilation	↓ Preload and afterload	Corrects pulmonary oedema ↑ Cardiac output
Inotropes Dobutamine (250–750 μg/min)	Sympathomimetic	↑ Contractility	↑ Cardiac output
Dopamine (100–600 μg/min)	Sympathomimetic	↑ Contractility ↓ Afterload (low dose) ↑ Afterload (high dose)	↑ Cardiac output ↑ Blood pressure (high dose)

Fig.92 Patients with acute LVF and pulmonary oedema often respond well to morphine and diuretics. Failure to respond rapidly to simple measures of this type is an indication for pulmonary artery pressure monitoring with a Swan Ganz catheter. Infusions of vasodilators and inotropes may then be given with the aim of adjusting the pulmonary artery wedge pressure to a level that allows pulmonary oedema to clear (15 to 18 mmHg) and increasing cardiac output to improve vital organ perfusion.

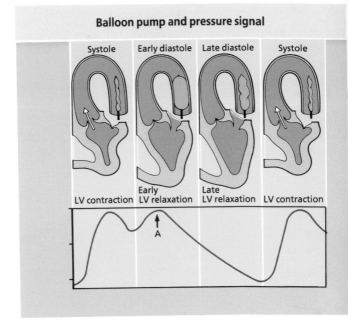

Balloon pump and pressure signal

Systole | Early diastole | Late diastole | Systole

LV contraction | Early LV relaxation | Late LV relaxation | LV contraction

Fig.93 Intra-aortic balloon pump and simultaneous aortic pressure signal. The balloon pump may be used to provide temporary support in severe heart failure. A catheter with a terminal sausage-shaped balloon is introduced into the femoral artery and positioned in the thoracic aorta as shown. Balloon pumping is synchronized with the ECG, with inflation in early diastole and deflation immediately before ventricular systole. Pressure in the aortic root is therefore augmented (A) in early diastole, improving coronary perfusion; the abrupt fall in pressure on deflation of the balloon reduces afterload and improves cardiac output.

Step	Treatment
	Treatment of chronic heart failure
1	Correct aggravating factors, e.g. arrhythmias, hypertension, valve disease
2	Introduce a thiazide diuretic, e.g. bendrofluazide 2.5–5 mg daily
3	Substitute a loop diuretic, e.g. frusemide 40–80 mg daily
4	Add an ACE inhibitor, e.g. captropril 12.5–25 mg tds
5	Add digoxin 62.5–500 mg daily
6	Consider heart transplantation

Fig.94 Treatment of chronic heart failure.

A step-wise approach to treatment is recommended. Diuretics improve salt and water overload and correct systemic pulmonary congestion. Thiazides are useful in mild failure but the more potent loop diuretics are required in advanced cases. As requirement for frusemide rises above 40-80 mg daily, an ACE inhibitor should be added. This improves cardiac output by vasodilatation, reducing muscle fatigue during exertion. The neurohormonal actions of ACE inhibitors may also improve long-term prognosis (See Fig. 82). In severe heart failure inotropic support with digoxin is helpful, but at this stage prognosis is very poor and heart transplantation should be considered.

VALVULAR HEART DISEASE

Aortic stenosis

Causes of aortic stenosis		
Calcific disease	Congenital bicuspid valve	Rheumatic disease

Fig.95 Causes of aortic stenosis. With the decline in rheumatic fever in this country, calcific AS – a degenerative process affecting the elderly – has become the commonest cause of AS. Congenital bicuspid valves often remain untroublesome until middle-age when calcification usually supervenes.

Clinical Presentation of Aortic Stenosis	
Angina	– ↑ O_2 demand of hypertrophied LV
Dyspnoea	– ↑ diastolic pressure in stiff (*noncompliant*) LV
Syncope	– *either* paroxysmal ventricular arrhythmias *or* exertional cerebral hypoperfusion
LVF	– contractile failure as ventricle dilates
Sudden death	– ventricular arrhythmias

Fig.96 Clinical presentation of aortic stenosis. Note that LVF is a late event which occurs when compensatory LV hypertrophy is no longer sufficient to maintain adequate flow across the stenosed valve. The LV dilates and irreversible impairment of contractile function occurs.

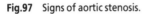

Signs of aortic disease

Auscultation at base of heart:
Ejection click (EC)
– if valve is mobile
Mid-systolic murmur (MSM)
– turbulent flow across
aortic valve

Carotid pulse:
slow upstroke, 'plateau'
pulse – reflects 'damped' LV
ejection across stenosed
aortic valve

LV impulse: thrusting
– reflects LV hypertrophy

S4: vigorous atrial
contraction to fill stiff,
'noncompliant' LV

Fig.97 Signs of aortic stenosis.

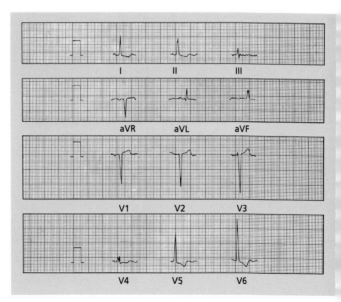

Fig.98 Aortic stenosis – ECG. Note the prominent voltage deflections in the chest leads (V$_1$ to V$_6$) associated with T wave inversion laterally (V$_5$ and V$_6$). This is a hypertrophy and strain pattern and is typical of conditions in which the LV is subjected to chronic pressure loading e.g. AS, hypertension. A similar pattern is seen in hypertrophic cardiomyopathy.

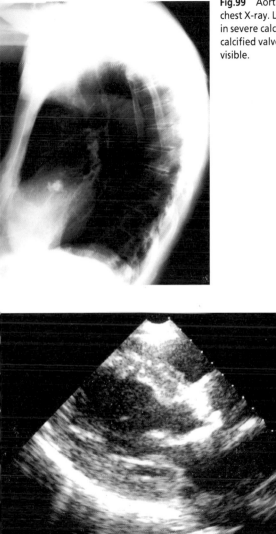

Fig.99 Aortic stenosis – chest X-ray. Lateral film in severe calcific AS. The calcified valve is clearly visible.

Fig.100 Aortic stenosis – echocardiogram. In this 2D study (long-axis view) the aortic valve is grossly thickened and highly echogenic. Concentric LV hypertrophy is present.

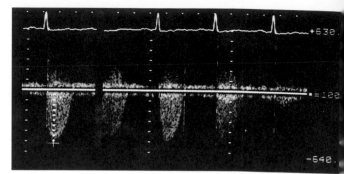

Fig.101 Aortic stenosis – Doppler echocardiography. The Doppler technique permits evaluation of the direction and velocity of flow within the heart and great vessels. Valvular stenosis causes the velocity (as opposed to volume) of flow across the valve to increase. This patient had severe aortic stenosis and the peak velocity of flow across the valve is 525 cm/sec, indicating a pressure gradient of 110 mmHg.

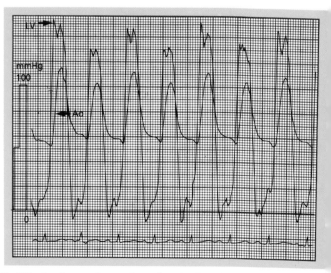

Fig.102 Aortic stenosis – cardiac catheterization. Simultaneous recordings of LV and aortic pressure signals. Note that LV pressure is higher than aortic pressure throughout systole. In this example *pulsus alternans* is present – a common finding in AS. The 'size' of the pressure gradient is determined by both the severity of the AS and the flow across the valve. In end stage disease the failing left ventricle is less able to generate pressure: flow across the valve declines and the gradient tends to fall.

Indications for valve replacement
1. Any symptoms of AS
2. ECG evidence of worsening LV hypertrophy and strain
3. Radiographic or echocardiographic evidence of LV dilatation and contractile failure
4. Peak systolic pressure gradient > 50mm Hg

Fig.103 Although AS is well tolerated for prolonged periods, the course is rapidly downhill after the development of symptoms with a three year survival of less than 50%. Irreversible deterioration of LV function is the principle cause of death. Aortic valve replacement corrects symptoms and improves prognosis considerably.

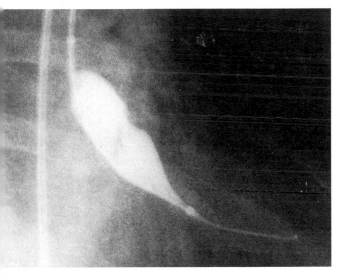

Fig.104 Aortic stenosis – balloon valvuloplasty. This new catherization technique is occasionally helpful in patients with aortic stenosis who are unfit for valve replacement surgery. A 20-25 mm balloon is inflated across the stenosed aortic valve in order to dilate it. Note the 'waisted' central portion of the balloon where it is compressed in the orifice of the diseased valve

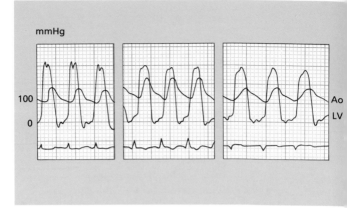

Fig.105 Aortic stenosis – balloon valvuloplasty, haemodynamic result. These are simultaneous recordings of the aortic (Ao) and LV pressure signals before (left), immediately after (centre), and three months after (right), aortic valvuloplasty. Before the procedure there is a substantial pressure gradient across the valve. Valvuloplasty successfully reduces the gradient but the benefit is only temporary and the gradient recurs after three months. This emphasises the limited value of this new technique which produces sustained improvement in very few patients.

Aortic regurgitation

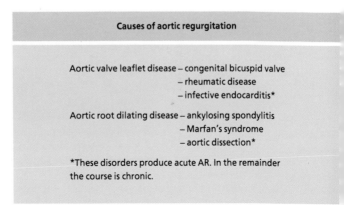

Causes of aortic regurgitation

Aortic valve leaflet disease – congenital bicuspid valve
– rheumatic disease
– infective endocarditis*

Aortic root dilating disease – ankylosing spondylitis
– Marfan's syndrome
– aortic dissection*

*These disorders produce acute AR. In the remainder the course is chronic.

Fig.106 Causes of aortic regurgitation.

Clinical presentation of aortic regurgitation	
Incidental finding	Mild to moderate AR is often asymptomatic
Angina	Increased oxygen demand of dilated hypertrophied LV
LVF	Contractile failure in advanced disease

Fig.107 Clinical presentation of aortic regurgitation.

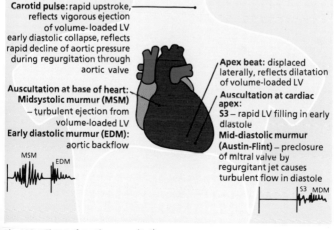

Signs of aortic regurgitation

Carotid pulse: rapid upstroke, reflects vigorous ejection of volume-loaded LV early diastolic collapse, reflects rapid decline of aortic pressure during regurgitation through aortic valve

Auscultation at base of heart: Midsystolic murmur (MSM) – turbulent ejection from volume-loaded LV
Early diastolic murmur (EDM): aortic backflow

MSM EDM

Apex beat: displaced laterally, reflects dilatation of volume-loaded LV
Auscultation at cardiac apex:
S3 – rapid LV filling in early diastole
Mid-diastolic murmur (Austin-Flint) – preclosure of mitral valve by regurgitant jet causes turbulent flow in diastole

S3 MDM

Fig.108 Signs of aortic regurgitation.

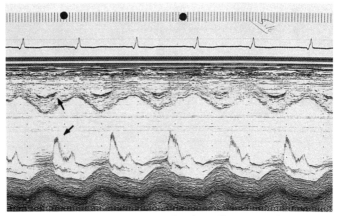

Fig.109 Aortic regurgitation – echocardiogram. M-mode echocardiogram in a patient who presented with acute aortic regurgitation. Dense vegetations (arrowed) are seen on the aortic valve. Gonococcus – a rare cause of endocarditis – was grown from blood cultures.

Fig.110 Aortic regurgitation – M-mode echocardiogram. Aortic regurgitation volume-loads the LV which is dilated but contracting vigorously. There is hypertrophy of the posterior wall. Note the fine vibrations on the interventricular septum and the anterior leaflet of the mitral valve (arrowed) caused by the regurgitant jet in early diastole.

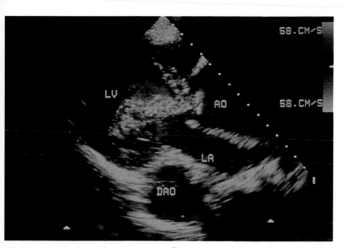

Fig.111 Aortic regurgitation – colour flow Doppler echocardiography. The direction of flow within the heart and great vessels is colour-coded, red indicating flow towards, and blue away from, the transducer. This patient has an aneurysm involving the ascending (Ao) and descending (DAo) aorta. There is a bright jet of aortic regurgitation extending beyond the anterior leaflet of the mitral valve towards the posterior wall of the LV.

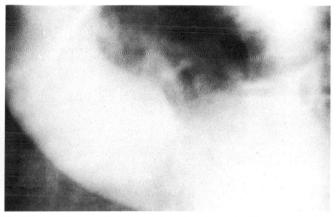

Fig.112 Aortic regurgitation – aortic root angiography. Contrast material has been injected into the ascending aorta through a catheter. Because the aortic valve is incompetent, rapid opacification of the left ventricular cavity has occurred. Note the dilatation of the proximal aorta – a typical finding in aortic valve disease.

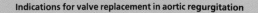

Indications for valve replacement in aortic regurgitation
1. Any symptoms of aortic regurgitation
2. Radiographic or echocardiographic evidence of worsening LV dilatation and contractile failure

Fig.113 Although the indications for valve replacement in aortic regurgitation are not clear cut, the procedure must be timed to prevent irreversible deterioration of LV contractile function.

Mitral Stenosis

Causes of mitral stenosis
Rheumatic disease
Congenital mitral stenosis

Fig.114 Causes of mitral stenosis. MS is nearly always a consequence of rheumatic disease.

Clinical presentation of mitral stenosis	
Dyspnoea, orthopnoea	– ↑ left atrial pressure
Right ventricular failure	– passive consequence of ↑ left atrial pressure and reactive pulmonary vasoconstriction
Palpitations	– atrial fibrillation
Systemic emboli	– atrial dilatation and fibrillation

Fig.115 Clinical presentation of mitral stenosis. Because of the risk of systemic emboli, atrial fibrillation in patients with mitral valve disease is an indication for anticoagulant therapy.

Signs of mitral stenosis

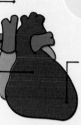

JVP: may be raised in RV failure ⟶

RV impulse: may be prominent in RV failure

Auscultation at cardiac apex:
Loud S1 – forceful closure of MV leaflets which are widely separated at the onset of systole
Opening snap (OS) in early diastole – forceful opening of MV due to increased LA pressure
Mid-diastolic murmur (MDM) with pre-systolic accentuation (PSA) in sinus rhythm – turbulent flow across mitral valve accentuated by atrial systole

Fig.116 Signs of mitral stenosis.

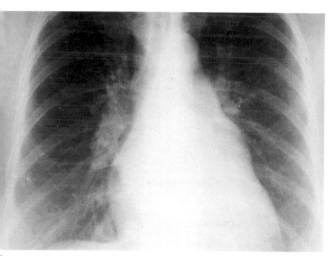

Fig.117 Mitral stenosis – chest X-ray. The enlarged left atrium produces a 'double contour' to the right heart border and prominence of the left heart border below the main pulmonary artery. Dilatation of the upper lobe pulmonary veins (reflecting elevated left atrial pressure) is clearly visible.

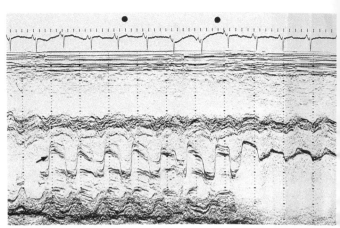

Fig.118 Mitral stenosis – M-mode echocardiogram. The aortic valve is normal but the mitral valve (arrowed) is thickened with dilatation of the left atrium.

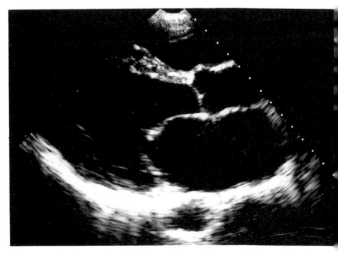

Fig.119 Mitral stenosis – 2D echocardiogram (long axis view – diastolic frame).The thickened mitral valve leaflets are poorly separated restricting flow across the valve. Raised pressure within the dilated atrium causes 'doming' of the mitral valve leaflets.

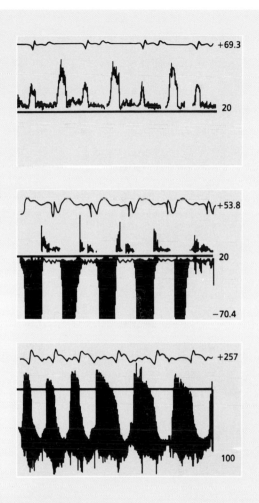

Fig.120 Doppler studies of mitral flow. Flow velocity is represented by the scale on the right side of each diagram.

Top. Normal mitral flow shows a biphasic pattern peaking in early diastole, immediately after the valve opens, and again in late diastole during atrial contraction.

Middle. In mitral regurgitation, the normal diastolic flow pattern is preserved but during systole a high velocity regurgitant jet is recorded.

Bottom. Mitral stenosis produces a high velocity jet in diastole. Atrial fibrillation ensures complete loss of the normal biphasic flow pattern.

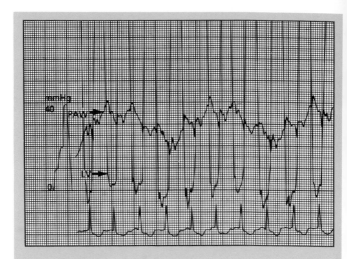

Fig.121 Mitral stenosis – cardiac catheterization. Simultaneous recordings of LV and pulmonary artery wedge (= left atrial) pressure signals. Note that left atrial pressure is higher than LV pressure throughout diastole. The rhythm is atrial fibrillation.

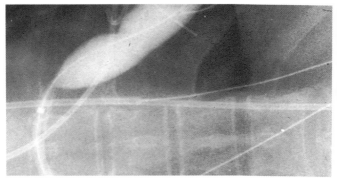

Fig.122 Mitral stenosis – balloon valvuloplasty. In patients with a non-calcified, competent (no regurgitation) valve this new technique is often very successful and avoids the need for heart surgery. The balloon catheter is advanced from the femoral vein into the right atrium and thence into the left atrium by trans-septal puncture. The balloon is positioned across the stenosed mitral valve and inflated as shown. Note the 'waisted' central portion of the balloon where it is compressed in the orifice of the diseased valve.

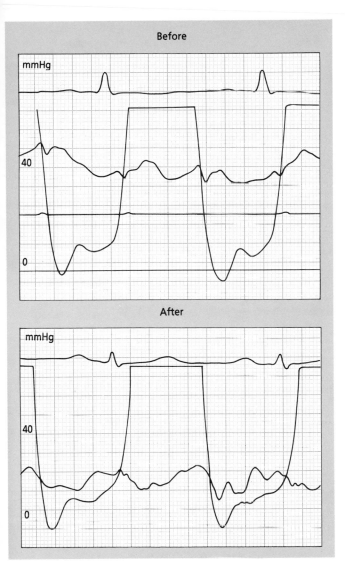

Before

After

Fig.123 Mitral stenosis – balloon valvuloplasty, haemodynamic result. These are simultaneous recordings of the PAWP and LV pressure signals before (left) and after (right) mitral valvuloplasty. Before the procedure there is a substantial pressure gradient across the valve. Valvuloplasty successfully reduces the gradient and can produce sustained benefit, unlike aortic valvuloplasty where improvement is often temporary (see Fig.105).

Mitral Regurgitation

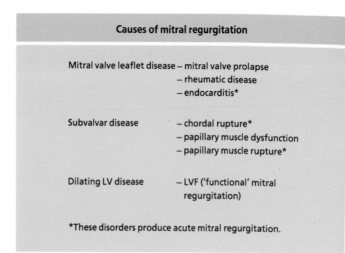

Causes of mitral regurgitation

Mitral valve leaflet disease – mitral valve prolapse
– rheumatic disease
– endocarditis*

Subvalvar disease – chordal rupture*
– papillary muscle dysfunction
– papillary muscle rupture*

Dilating LV disease – LVF ('functional' mitral
regurgitation)

*These disorders produce acute mitral regurgitation.

Fig.124 Causes of mitral regurgitation.

Clinical presentation of mitral regurgitation

Dyspnoea – ↑ left atrial pressure, particularly during
exertion

LVF – contractile failure with severe
ventricular dilatation

RVF – passive consequence of ↑ left atrial
pressure

Systemic emboli – atrial dilatation and fibrillation.

Fig.125 Clinical presentation of mitral regurgitation. Note that frank LVF
is a late event in chronic mitral regurgitation. Because of the risk of systemic
emboli, atrial fibrillation in patients with mitral valve disease is an
indication for anticoagulant therapy.

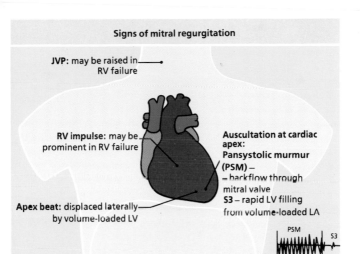

Signs of mitral regurgitation

JVP: may be raised in RV failure

RV impulse: may be prominent in RV failure

Auscultation at cardiac apex:
Pansystolic murmur (PSM) –
– backflow through mitral valve
S3 – rapid LV filling from volume-loaded LA

Apex beat: displaced laterally by volume-loaded LV

PSM   S3

Fig.126 Signs of mitral regurgitation.

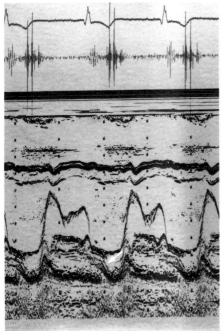

Fig.127 Mitral valve prolapse. This is a common and usually asymptomatic condition. The cause is often unknown but it may be associated with many cardiac and systemic disorders. Systolic prolapse of one or both valve leaflets into the left atrium produces a click and a variable degree of MR. The echocardiogram shows systolic prolapse of the posterior mitral leaflet (arrowed). The click and murmur have been recorded on the phonocardiogram. In this case two additional clicks of greater intensity occur later in systole.

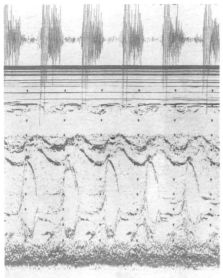

Fig.128 Mitral regurgitation – M-mode echocardiogram with simultaneous phonocardiogram in a patient with chordal rupture and severe MR. The pansystolic murmur has been recorded on the phonocardiogram. Note the wide excursion of the mitral valve leaflets during diastole, and the vigorous contraction of the somewhat dilated LV.

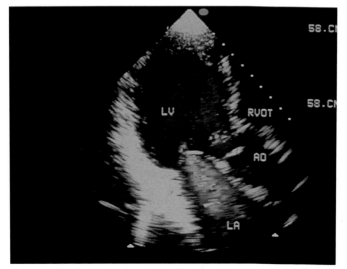

Fig.129 Mitral regurgitation – colour flow Doppler echocardiography. This is an apical long-axis view of the heart showing a large jet of mitral regurgitation (blue) occupying most of the left atrial cavity (LA).

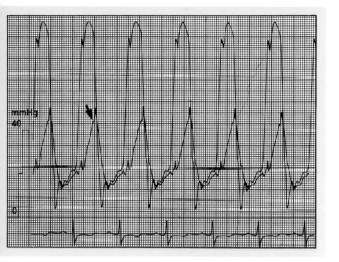

Fig.130 Cardiac catheterization in severe MR. Simultaneous recordings of LV and PAW (= left atrial) pressure signals. During systole, mitral backflow produces a rapid rise in left atrial pressure as reflected by the giant 'V' wave (arrowed) on the wedge trace.

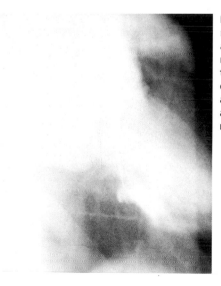

Fig.131 Mitral regurgitation – LV angiogram. Contrast material injected into the left ventricle rapidly opacifies the dilated left atrium due to backflow across the diseased mitral valve.

Mitral valve disease – indications for surgery and choice of surgical procedure	
Symptoms	– effort-related dyspnoea not controlled by therapy
Catheter findings	– significant mitral stenosis (exercise gradient >12 mmHg) – significant mitral regurgitation
Surgical procedures	– commisurotomy for 'pure' mitral stenosis in the absence of calcification and significant subvalvar disease – valve replacement for other cases of mitral stenosis and all cases of mitral regurgitation

Fig.132 Indications for mitral valve surgery.

Tricuspid and pulmonary valve disease

Causes of tricuspid and pulmonary valve disease	
Pulmonary stenosis	– congenital – rheumatic (rare)
Pulmonary regurgitation	– pulmonary hypertension – infective endocarditis
Tricuspid stenosis	– rheumatic
Tricuspid regurgitation	– 'functional' – infective endocarditis – rheumatic

Fig.133 Disease of the pulmonary and tricuspid valve is a rare cause of right ventricular failure. Indeed, tricuspid regurgitation – the commonest right sided valve lesion – is nearly always a secondary consequence of right ventricular failure, which itself is usually caused by left heart failure or pulmonary vascular disease. Primary pulmonary and tricuspid disease can lead to right-sided failure manifested by systemic congestion and low cardiac output.

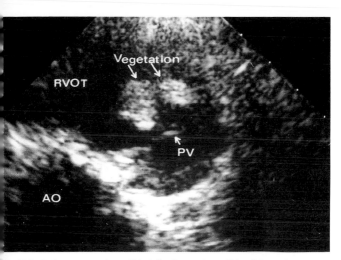

Fig.134 Pulmonary endocarditis. Infective endocarditis of the pulmonary and tricuspid valves is unusual and occurs most commonly in intravenous drug abusers. In this 2D echocardiogram large vegetations are seen on the pulmonary valve (PV). The aorta (AO) and the right ventricular outflow tract (RVOT) are shown.

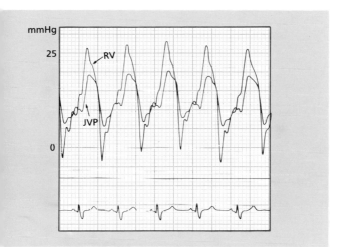

Fig.135 Tricuspid regurgitation. Simultaneous recordings of the right ventricular (RV) and jugular venous pressure (JVP). Note the giant 'v' waves in the JVP during RV systole caused by regurgitation through the tricuspid valve.

MYOCARDIAL AND PERICARDIAL DISEASE

Cardiomyopathy	
Definition	A chronic heart muscle disorder of unknown cause
Classification	
Dilated cardiomyopathy	Ventricular dilatation and hypertrophy with global impairment of systolic contraction
Hypertrophic cardiomyopathy	Ventricular hypertrophy with global impairment of diastolic relaxation
Restrictive cardiomyopathy	Endomyocardial fibrosis with global impairment of diastolic relaxation (common in the tropics but rarely seen in the UK)

Fig.136 Cardiomyopathy.

Specific heart muscle disease		
Systolic dysfunction	**Diastolic dysfunction**	**Diastolic dysfunction**
(physiology similar to dilated cardiomyopathy	(physiology similar to hypertrophic cardiomyopathy)	(physiology similar to restrictive cardiomyopathy)
Coronary artery disease	Hypertension	Amyloidosis
Viral myocarditis	Aortic stenosis	
Alcoholic heart disease	Freidrich's ataxia	
Daunorubicin toxicity		
Muscular dystrophy		
Diabetes		

Fig.137 Specific heart muscle disease. These disorders may all cause (or be associated with) specific heart muscle disease which is often clinically indistinguishable from cardiomyopathy. The differential diagnosis is important, however, because in some cases correction of the underlying disorders prevents progression of the heart disease.

Dilated Cardiomyopathy

Clinical presentation of dilated cardiomyopathy
1. Heart failure
2. Systemic and pulmonary embolism
3. Sudden death
4. Non-specific ECG abnormalities
5. Cardiac enlargement and variable pulmonary congestion on the chest X-ray

Fig.138 Clinical presentation of dilated cardiomyopathy.

Dilated cardiomyopathy usually presents with biventricular failure. Mural thrombi are common within the dilated cardiac chamber and predispose to systemic and pulmonary embolism. These patients are prone to atrial and ventricular arrhythmias and may die suddenly. The ECG and chest X-ray are nearly always abnormal. Physical signs are those of congestive heart failure (see Fig.83).

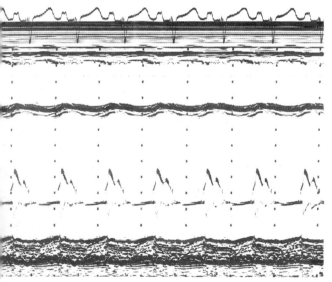

Fig.139 Echocardiogram. The LV cavity is dilated with severly impaired septal and posterior wall contractile function. The patient had idiopathic congestive cardiomyopathy and later underwent successful heart transplantation.

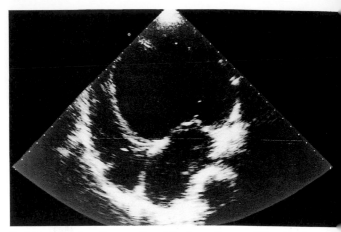

Fig.140 Dilated cardiomyopathy – 2D echocardiogram. This apical four-chamber view shows gross dilatation of the left ventricle and left atrium with global contractile impairment.

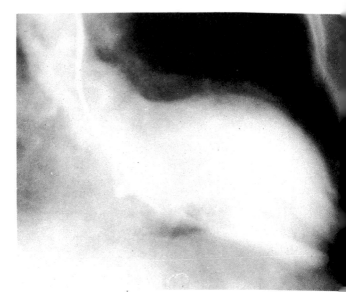

Fig.141 Dilated cardiomyopathy – LV angiogram. This is a systolic frame showing a very dilated poorly contractile LV.

Hypertrophic cardiomyopathy

Clinical presentation of hypertrophic cardiomyopathy	
1. Angina	Increased LV muscle mass
2. Heart failure	Impaired LV relaxation in diastole
3. Sudden death	Ventricular arrhythmias
4. Abnormal ECG	Exaggerated voltage deflections of LV hypertrophy

Fig.142 Clinical presentation of hypertrophic cardiomyopathy.

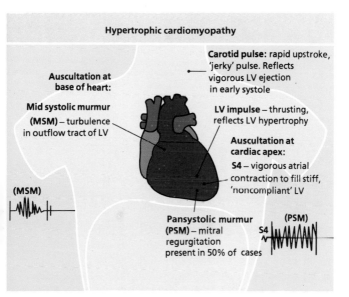

Fig.143 Physical examination in hypertrophic cardiomyopathy.

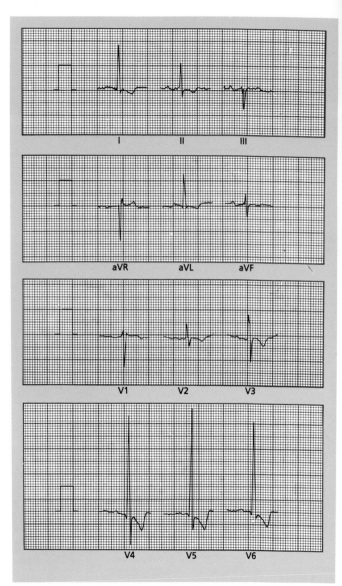

Fig.144 Hypertrophic cardiomyopathy – ECG. The ECG is nearly always abnormal in hypertrophic cardiomyopathy with exaggerated voltage deflections and T wave changes reflecting LV hypertrophy.

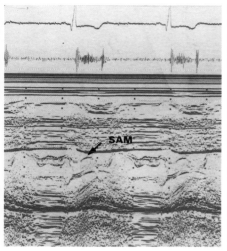

Fig.145 Hypertrophic cardiomyopathy – echocardiogram. Note the massive septal hypertrophy (3mm) with normal posterior wall thickness. Systolic anterior movement (SAM) of the anterior mitral valve leaflet (arrowed) is a typical feature of the condition and contributes to the outflow tract obstruction. The ejection systolic murmur recorded on the phonocardiogram reflects turbulence in the obstructed LV outflow tract.

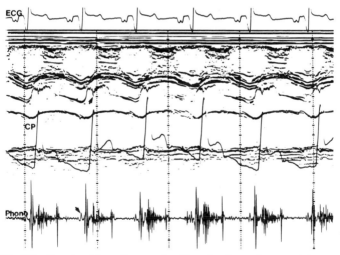

Fig.146 Hypertrophic cardiomyopathy. M-mode echocardiogram of the aortic valve with simultaneous carotid pulse (CP) recording and phonocardiogram. Note the sharp upstroke to the carotid pulse with an abrupt decline in midsystole associated with premature closure of the aortic valve (arrowed) – an important feature of hypertrophic cardiomyopathy. The phonocardiogram shows the fourth heart sound (arrowed) and the systolic ejection murmur characteristic of the condition.

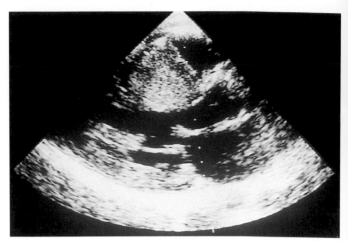

Fig.147 Hypertrophic cardiomyopathy – 2D-echocardiogram. This long-axis view shows gross LV hypertrophy, particularly involving the interventricular septum and the papillary muscles.

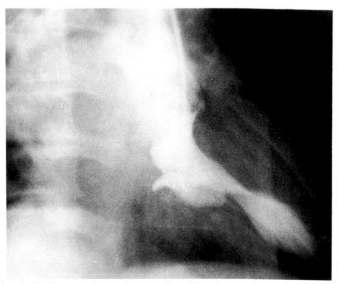

Fig.148 Hypertrophic cardiomyopathy – LV angiogram. Although diastolic relaxation is severely impaired in hypertrophic cardiomyopathy, systolic contraction is usually hyperdynamic. In this systolic frame there is almost total obliteration of the LV cavity in the outflow tract below the aortic valve.

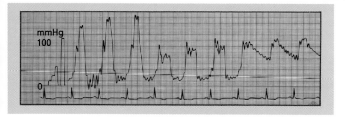

Fig.149 Hypertrophic cardiomyopathy – LV outflow gradient. The systolic anterior motion of the mitral valve and the hyperdynamic LV contraction (Figs 145 and 148) may combine to produce a subvalvar pressure gradient. The illustration shows pressure recordings during pull back of a catheter from the apex of the LV to the aorta. There is a systolic pressure gradient (75 mmHg) at subvalvar level in the LV outflow tract but not across the valve itself.

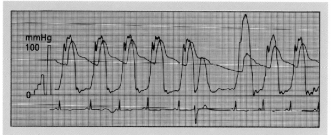

Fig.150 Hypertrophic cardiomyopathy – provocation of LV outflow gradient, ventricular premature beat. The outflow tract obstruction in hypertrophic cardiomyopathy is 'dynamic' unlike the valvular obstruction in aortic stenosis which is 'fixed'. Various manoeuvres will provoke an outflow tract gradient. Here, simultaneous recordings of LV and aortic pressure signals show provocation of a gradient in the beat following a VPB.

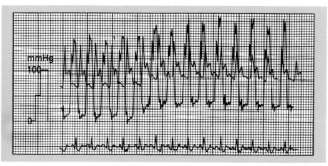

Fig.151 Hypertrophic cardiomyopathy – provocation of LV outflow tract obstruction, Valsalva manoeuvre. Simultaneous recordings of the LV and aortic pressure signals before and during the Valsalva manoeuvre.

Pericardial Disease

Acute pericarditis

Causes of acute pericarditis

1. Idiopathic

2. Infective – viral (Coxsackie B, influenza, herpes)
   – bacterial (*Staphylococcus aureus*)
     Mycobacterium tuberculosis)

3. Connective tissue disease – systemic lupus,
     rheumatoid arthritis

4. Uraemia

5. Malignancy – breast, lung, lymphoma, leukaemia

6. Radiation therapy

7. Post myocardial infarction/cardiotomy
     – Dressler's syndrome

Fig.152 Causes of acute pericarditis.

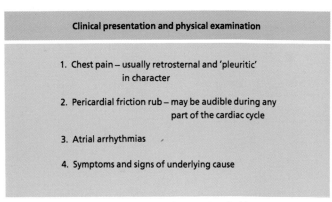

Clinical presentation and physical examination

1. Chest pain – usually retrosternal and 'pleuritic'
     in character

2. Pericardial friction rub – may be audible during any
     part of the cardiac cycle

3. Atrial arrhythmias

4. Symptoms and signs of underlying cause

Fig.153 Any cause of pericarditis may be associated with pericardial effusion. If the effusion is large the heart sounds may be diminished in intensity. A pericardial friction rub does not preclude the presence of a large effusion.

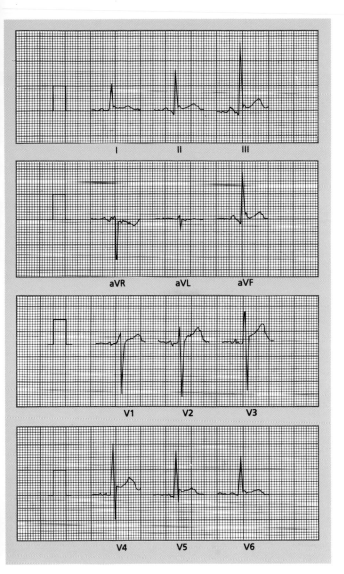

Fig.154 Pericarditis – ECG. In pericarditis, minor subepicardial injury produces ST segment elevation affecting any or all of the ECG leads (except aVR) depending on the site of pericardial inflammation. The elevated ST segments are characteristically concave upwards and return towards the baseline as the pericardial inflammation subsides.

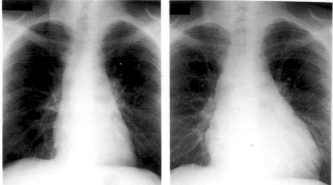

Fig.155 Tuberculous pericarditis. The patient presented with a history of fever and recent retrosternal pleuritic pain. The chest X-ray showed enlarged hilar lymph nodes (left). Cervical lymph node biopsy subsequently confirmed tuberculosis. Two weeks later the heart size was significantly larger due to pericardial effusion.

Cardiac tamponade

Clinical presentation and physical examination
1. Low output state – hypotension, oliguria, cold periphery
2. Tachycardia
3. Pulsus paradoxus
4. ↑ JVP with rapid 'X' descent
5. Kussmaul's sign – paradoxical rise in JVP with deep inspiration
6. 'Distant' heart sounds

Fig.156 Any cause of pericardial effusion can produce tamponade depending on the size of the effusion and the rapidity with which it develops. The gradual accumulation of pericardial fluid permits progressive stretching of the pericardial sac such that substantial effusions may develop without significant increments in intrapericardial pressure. Rapid accumulations of fluid, on the other hand, lead to critical elevation of pressure within the pericardial sac. This restricts ventricular filling and causes marked reduction in cardiac output. Urgent pericardiocentesis is mandatory in cardiac tamponade.

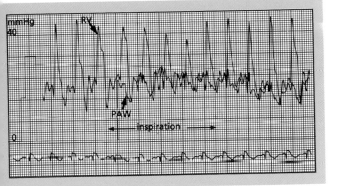

Fig.157 Tamponade – pathophysiology. In tamponade, intrapericardial pressure rises and restricts cardiac filling. The thin-walled RV is worst affected. A compensatory rise in RV filling pressure occurs which comes to equal LV filling pressure. Thereafter, filling pressures of both ventricles rise together as tamponade increases. This illustration shows simultaneous recordings of the RV and pulmonary artery wedge (PAW) pressures in severe tamponade.

Note: 1. Equalization and elevation of RV diastolic and PAW pressures (the right and left ventricular filling pressures, respectively).
2. During inspiration RV filling pressure *increases* (Kussmaul's sign) and peak systolic pressure declines (pulsus paradoxus).

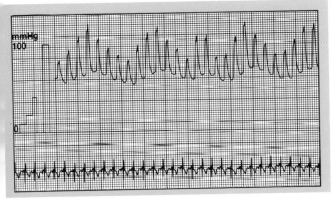

Fig.158 Tamponade – pulsus paradoxus. Radial artery pressure recording in cardiac tamponade. Note the exaggerated decline in arterial pressure during inspiration. Pulsus paradoxus is nearly always present in tamponade but may also occur in constrictive pericarditis, severe obstructive airways disease and tension pneumothorax.

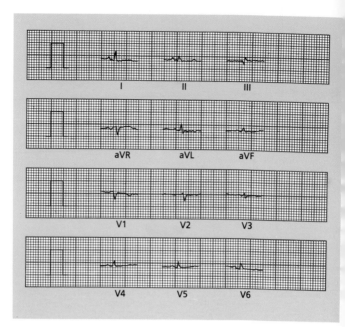

Fig.159 Tamponade – ECG. The voltage deflections in cardiac tamponade are usually of low amplitude due to the insulating effect of the pericardial effusion.

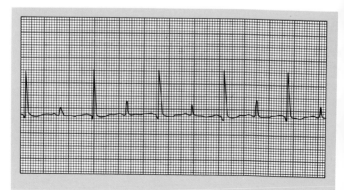

Fig.160 Tamponade – electrical alternans. This is a relatively unusual ECG manifestation of pericardial effusion and tamponade. The beat to beat variation in R wave magnitude reflects an alternating electrical axis caused by unrestricted movement of the heart within the fluid-filled pericardial sac.

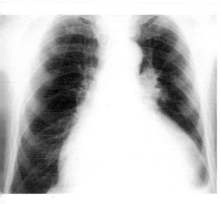

Fig.161 Tamponade. The chest X-ray shows a left hilar mass caused by cancer. Pericardial infiltration has produced effusion and tamponade evidenced by the severe cardiac enlargement. Malignant disease is now the most common cause of tamponade in this country.

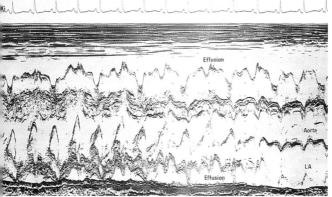

Fig.162 Tamponade and electrical alternans. The m-mode echocardiogram shows an echo-free space in front of and behind the heart caused by pericardial effusion. Note the electrical alternans on the ECG.

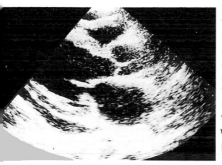

Fig.163 Tamponade. The 2D-echocardiogram (long-axis view) shows an echo-free space around the heart. The effusion is small, but in this case developed rapidly and was sufficient to cause tamponade within the noncompliant pericardial sac.

Constrictive pericarditis

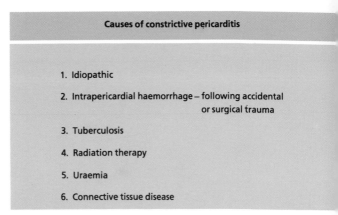

Causes of constrictive pericarditis

1. Idiopathic
2. Intrapericardial haemorrhage – following accidental or surgical trauma
3. Tuberculosis
4. Radiation therapy
5. Uraemia
6. Connective tissue disease

Fig.164 Constrictive pericarditis may follow *any* acute pericardial injury. Tuberculosis is no longer the commonest cause in this country where most cases are either idiopathic or the result of intrapericardial haemorrhage following heart surgery.

Clinical presentation and physical examination

1. Oedema and ascites
2. ↑ JVP with rapid 'X' and 'Y' descents
3. Kussmaul's sign
4. Pericardial knock on auscultation
5. Pulsus paradoxus (unusual)

Fig.165 Constrictive pericarditis is a chronic wasting illness. Fibrosis and shrinkage of the pericardial sac restricts ventricular filling despite progressive elevation and equilibration of the ventricular filling pressures. Although symptoms and signs of low cardiac output may be present, the consequences of elevated systemic venous pressure and salt and water retention dominate the clinical picture. Treatment is by surgical excision of the pericardium.

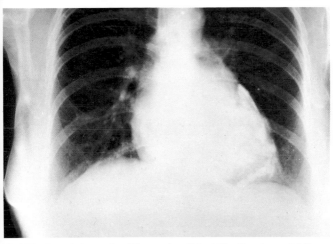

Fig.166 Constrictive pericarditis – pericardial calcification. In constrictive pericarditis, pericardial calcification is seen in less than 50% of cases. Here it is seen clearly on the postero-anterior chest X-ray, but the lateral projection is usually more useful.

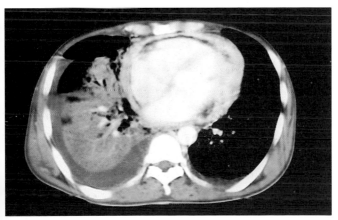

Fig.167 Constrictive pericarditis computed tomography There is consolidation in the right lung and severe pericardial thickening. The patient had pulmonary tuberculosis with pericardial involvement and presented with fever and signs of constriction. Antituberculous therapy caused regression of all symptoms and signs although the patient is at major risk of developing constriction later as the pericardium becomes fibrotic and calcified.

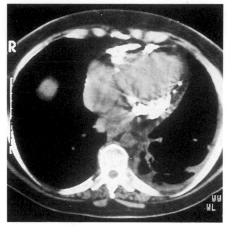

Fig.168 Constrictive pericarditis – computed tomography. There is dense calcification of the pericardium which is white with an appearance similar to bone. The patient had had tuberculosis several years previously.

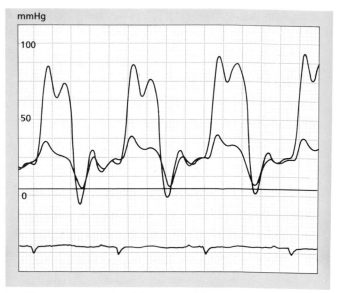

Fig.169 Constrictive pericarditis – left and right ventricular pressure signals. Constriction affects both ventricles equally and the diastolic pressures must rise and equilibrate to maintain ventricular filling (cf tamponade). Thus in diastole the pressure signals are superimposed with a typical 'dip and plateau' configuration.

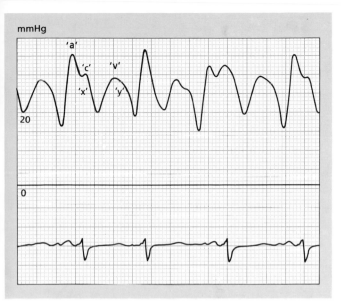

Fig.170 Constrictive pericarditis – right atrial pressure signal. The pressure is elevated, and prominence of the 'x' descent (interrupted by the 'c' wave) and the 'y' descent is clearly visible. These waves are not easy to identify clinically but they give the JVP an unusually dynamic appearance.

CARDIAC ARRHYTHMIAS

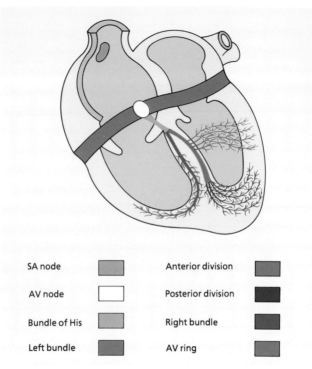

SA node		Anterior division	
AV node		Posterior division	
Bundle of His		Right bundle	
Left bundle		AV ring	

Fig.171 Normal conducting pathways. Synchronized contraction of the four cardiac chambers depends on the highly organized spread of a wave of depolarization throughout the heart. All cardiac cells exhibit the property of **excitability** whereby a stimulus of sufficient magnitude produces rapid membrane depolarization followed by a slower repolarization process. Only the specialized conducting tissues, however, can depolarize spontaneously under normal circumstances. This property which is called **automaticity** is essential to the pacemaker function of the sinus node – the conducting tissue with the highest intrinsic firing rate. The impulse generated by the sinus node spreads first through the atria producing atrial systole and then through the atrioventricular (AV) node to the His-Purkinje system producing ventricular systole. Impulse conduction through the AV node is slow and cannot proceed above a certain rate. This ensures that:
1. There is adequate delay between atrial and ventricular systole for optimal cardiac performance.
2. The ventricles are protected from having to respond to very rapid atrial rhythms.

Mechanisms of arrhythmias

1. *Automatic mechanisms.* A variety of stimuli – including trauma, ischaemia and drug toxicity – can enhance the automaticity of the conducting tissue below the sinus node and produce isolated premature beats. Automaticity can also be acquired by damaged or diseased cells otherwise not capable of impulse generation. Repeated automatic discharge from an 'ectopic' focus of this type at a rate in excess of the sinus node (or any other established pacemaker) can take over the pacemaker function of the heart and result in atrial or ventricular tachyarrhythmias.

2. *Re-entry mechanisms.* The basic requirements for re-entry are the coexistence of unidirectional block to impulse traffic in part of the conducting system and retrograde conduction via an alternative pathway. This permits the establishment of a re-entry circuit in response to premature stimuli. Re-entry mechanisms are probably responsible for the majority of sustained atrial and ventricular tachyarrhythmias.

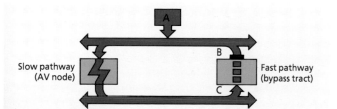

Fig.172 A re-entry circuit. This figure illustrates a typical re-entry circuit involving the AV node and a fast conducting bypass tract. A premature atrial impulse (A) is blocked at point B in the fast pathway but conducts through the AV node. Thereafter rapid ventricular depolarization occurs via His-Purkinje pathways and cells immediately distal to the block (point C) are activated. By now the bypass tract is no longer refractory and conducts the impulse retrogradely into the atria thereby completing the re-entry circuit and initiating self-sustaining circus movement. The Wolff-Parkinson-White syndrome (Figs. 188-191) provides a useful model for re-entry arrhythmias.

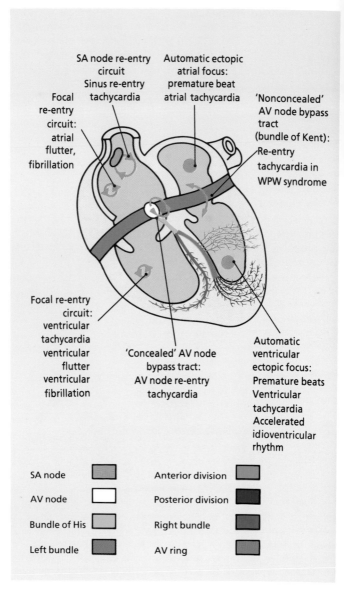

Fig.173 Mechanism of arrhythmias. Automatic ectopic foci and re-entry circuits are the pathophysiological substrate for all the common cardiac arrhythmias.

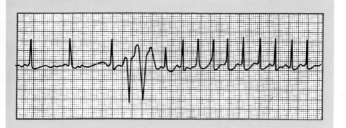

Fig.174 Sinus node re-entry tachycardia. Sinus rhythm is interrupted by a couplet of ventricular premature beats which triggers the tachycardia. Note that the P wave – QRS relationship is unaffected by the tachycardia because it originates within the sinus node.

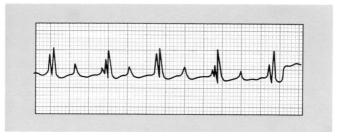

Fig.175 Atrial tachycardia with AV block. The atrial rate is 210/min but the ventricular rate is slower because of AV block. Note that AV block causes dissociation of the P waves from the QRS complexes.

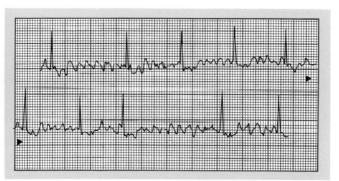

Fig.176 Established AF. Coarse fibrillatory waves are clearly seen with a controlled ventricular response.

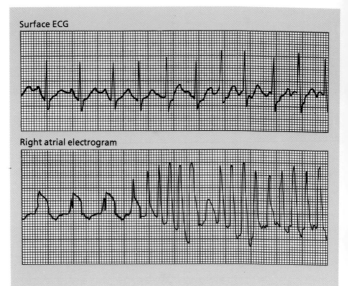

Fig.177 Atrial fibrillation. The fibrillatory waves are not always so clearly visible as in Fig.176. In this example, sinus rhythm gives way to an irregular tachycardia (rate about 150/min) after the third beat. A simultaneous right atrial electrogram – recorded from within the right atrial cavity – shows an irregular fibrillatory pattern (rate about 400/min) which confirms the diagnosis of atrial fibrillation.

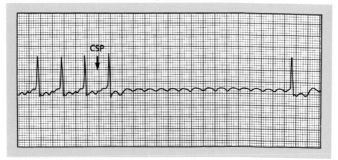

Fig.178 Atrial flutter. The ventricular rate is 150/min which is highly suggestive of atrial flutter with 2:1 AV block. However, not until AV block is increased by the application of carotid sinus pressure (CSP) do the flutter waves becomes apparent at a rate of 300/min.

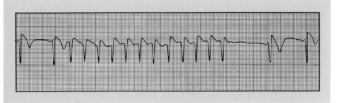

Fig.179 Paroxysmal AV nodal re-entry tachycardia. After the second sinus beat an atrial premature beat initiates a self-limiting paroxysm of tachycardia. Note that the QRS complexes are narrow and morphologically identical to the QRS complexes during sinus rhythm. This confirms the supraventricular origin of the arrhythmia.

Differential diagnosis of broad complex tachycardias		
	Supraventricular tachycardia	Ventricular tachycardia
QRS morphology		
QRS width	< 140 ms	> 140 ms
RBBB pattern V1	rSR′ with R′ > r	RSr′ with R > r′
V6		QS or RS with S > R
AV relationship		
P-QRS ratio	≥ 1:1	≤ 1:1
P-QRS relationship	Associated	Dissociated
		– independent P waves
		– fusion/capture beats
12 lead ECG		
Frontal plane QRS axis	Normal	Left (< −30°)
Rhythm Strip		
QRS deflections	Concordant	Shifting wave fronts (torsades)

Fig.180 Differential diagnosis of broad complex tachycardias. This may be difficult and if possible a rhythm strip and a 12 lead ECG should be obtained. The findings in this table provide a useful diagnostic guide.

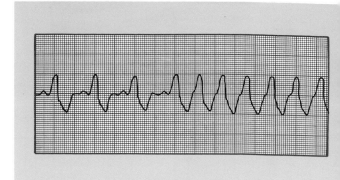

Fig.181 Broad complex tachycardia – supraventricular or ventricular? After the fourth sinus beat there is a broad complex tachycardia. Note, however, that the sinus complexes are themselves broad and morphologically identical to the tachycardia complexes. This strongly suggests a supraventricular origin of the arrhythmia.

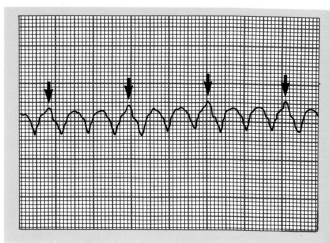

Fig.182 Atrioventricular dissociation. In this example P waves (arrowed) can be seen 'marching through' the VT indicating that the atrial and ventricular rhythms are dissociated and that the broad complexes are ventricular in origin.

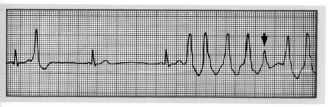

Fig.183 Atrioventricular dissociation – ventricular capture or fusion beats. During the VT the dissociated atrial rhythm will occasionally penetrate the AV node and produce either a normal QRS complex (capture) or, more commonly, a hybrid complex representing fusion of the sinus and ventricular beats. In this example, VT is initiated by a very early VPB (morphologically similar to the previous isolated VPB) and is interrupted by a fusion beat (arrowed) confirming the ventricular origin of the tachycardia.

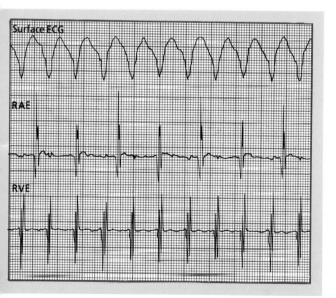

Fig.184 If atrioventricular dissociation is not clear on the surface ECG, simultaneous recordings of the electrograms from within the right atrium (RAE) and right ventricle (RVE) can be helpful. Here the broad complex tachycardia on the surface ECG is simultaneous with the deflections on the RVE, but the deflections on the RAE are slower and bear no fixed relation to the complexes on the surface ECG. This indicates atrioventricular dissociation and confirms the ventricular origin of the tachycardia.

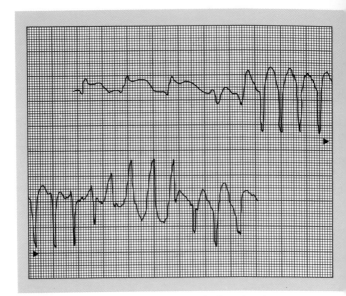

Fig.185 Torsades de pointes. In this example three sinus beats are followed by a broad complex tachycardia. The changing wave fronts (torsades de pointes) during the tachycardia confirm it is ventricular in origin.

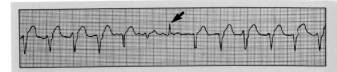

Fig.186 Accelerated idioventricular rhythm. Ventricular rhythms with a rate of 60 to 120 beats/min are included in this category. The arrhythmia rarely occurs except in the context of acute myocardial infarction. The slow ventricular automatic focus is usually in continuous competition with the sinus node such that the idioventricular rhythm is typically episodic and alternates with episodes of sinus rhythm. Specific therapy is not necessary since the ventricular rate is not, by definition, fast and haemodynamic stability is usually well maintained. In this example the idioventricular rhythm is interrupted by 'fusion' beats (part sinus and part idioventricular in origin) and a single sinus beat (arrowed).

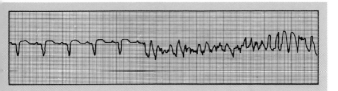

Fig.187 Ventricular fibrillation. This is a completely disorganized ventricular rhythm characterized by irregular fibrillatory waves with no discernible QRS complexes. VF is incompatible with an effective cardiac output and leads rapidly to death. Urgent treatment is therefore essential. In this example sinus rhythm terminates abruptly with the onset of VF. The patient was undergoing outpatient ambulatory monitoring of the ECG and died suddenly at home.

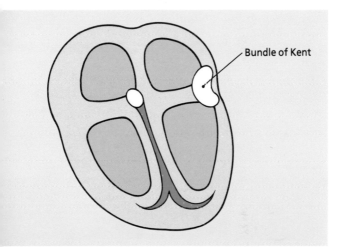

Bundle of Kent

Fig.188 Wolff-Parkinson-White syndrome: the anatomical substrate. Under normal circumstances AV conduction can proceed only via the AV node. The remainder of the AV ring tissue (see Fig.171) will not conduct impulse traffic. In Wolff-Parkinson-White syndrome, however, a congenital anomalous conduction pathway (bundle of Kent) exists between the atria and ventricles. Atrial impulses conduct more rapidly through the bundle of Kent than through the AV node and produce early ventricular activation or pre-excitation.

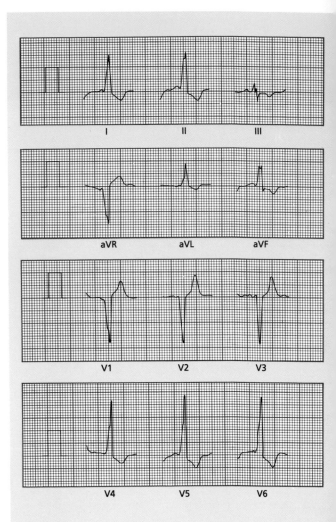

Fig.189 Wolff-Parkinson-White syndrome. The surface ECG. Ventricular pre-excitation is reflected on the surface ECG by a short PR interval and a slurred proximal limb of the QRS complex – the delta wave. The remainder of the QRS complex is usually normal because the delayed arrival of the impulse conducted through the AV node rapidly completes ventricular depolarization through normal His-Purkinje pathways.

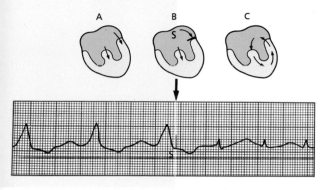

Fig.190 Wolff-Parkinson-White syndrome: re-entry tachycardia (recorded at fast paper speed). Just after the 3rd preexcited complex a premature atrial pacing stimulus (S) initiates an impulse that is blocked in the bundle of Kent but is conducted normally through the AV node producing ventricular depolarization *without* pre-excitation. Thus the QRS complex is narrow and lacks a delta wave. The impulse is conducted retrogradely through the bundle of Kent, re-enters that proximal conducting system, and completes the re-entry circuit, initiating self-sustaining re-entry tachycardia (last 3 complexes).

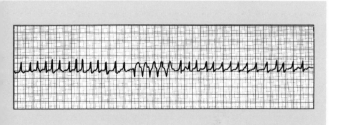

Fig.191 Wolff-Parkinson-White syndrome – atrial fibrillation. This is life-threatening if the bundle of Kent is able to conduct the rapid fibrillatory rhythm and produce a very rapid ventricular response of 300 beats/min or more. The risk of this degenerating into lethal ventricular fibrillation is high. Most patients, however, are protected from this because the bundle of Kent becomes refractory as the atrial rate increases and either fails to conduct in atrial fibrillation or conducts only intermittently. In this example there is intermittent conduction of atrial fibrillation by the bundle of Kent producing a short run of broad, pre-excited ventricular complexes. This poses no threat to the patient.

Detection of paroxysmal cardiac arrhythmias	
1. Ambulatory ('Holter') ECG monitoring	Useful if arrhythmia occurs frequently
2. Patient-activated ECG recording	Useful if arrhythmia is symptomatic but infrequent
3. Exercise ECG	Occasionally useful for exertional arrhythmias
4. In-hospital ECG monitoring	For high-risk patients who have had out of hospital cardiac arrest
5. Programmed cardiac stimulation	Electrode catheters directed into the heart permit electrical stimulation of arrhythmias and evaluation of the response to treatment

Fig.192   Detection of paroxysmal cardiac arrhythmias. ECG documentation of cardiac arrhythmias is an essential prerequisite to effective treatment. In patients with paroxysmal arrhythmias this may be difficult. The most widely used method is 24-hour Holter monitoring, but if attacks are infrequent a patient-activated recorder may be needed. The patient applies the device to the chest wall during an attack of palpitations and records the cardiac rhythm. The exercise ECG is not often helpful for arrhythmia detection and in difficult cases programmed cardiac stimulation is required.

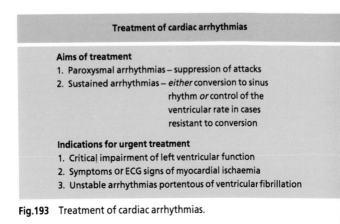

Treatment of cardiac arrhythmias

Aims of treatment
1. Paroxysmal arrhythmias – suppression of attacks
2. Sustained arrhythmias – *either* conversion to sinus rhythm *or* control of the ventricular rate in cases resistant to conversion

Indications for urgent treatment
1. Critical impairment of left ventricular function
2. Symptoms or ECG signs of myocardial ischaemia
3. Unstable arrhythmias portentous of ventricular fibrillation

Fig.193   Treatment of cardiac arrhythmias.

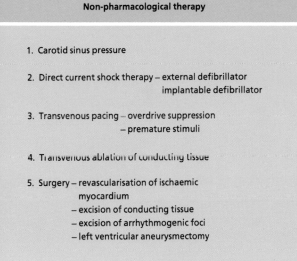

Non-pharmacological therapy

1. Carotid sinus pressure

2. Direct current shock therapy – external defibrillator
   implantable defibrillator

3. Transvenous pacing – overdrive suppression
   – premature stimuli

4. Transvenous ablation of conducting tissue

5. Surgery – revascularisation of ischaemic
   myocardium
   – excision of conducting tissue
   – excision of arrhythmogenic foci
   – left ventricular aneurysmectomy

194 Nonpharmacological treatment of cardiac arrhythmias. DC shock with an external defibrillator should not be delayed in patients with rapid, life-threatening arrhythmias. The internal defibrillator (implanted surgically) is being used increasingly for the treatment of life-threatening ventricular arrhythmias resistant to medical therapy.

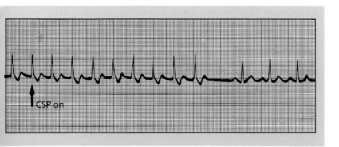

195 Carotid sinus pressure (CSP). Gentle massage of the carotid sinus produces a reflex increase in vagal discharge. This abruptly slows conduction through the AV node. The manoeuvre is useful for evaluation of the ECG during atrial flutter (see Fig. 178). On occasions CSP will break AV nodal re-entry circuits and convert SVT to sinus rhythm – as illustrated in this figure.

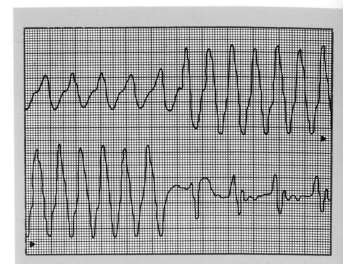

Fig.196 Burst overdrive pacing. This technique can be used for treatment of atrial or ventricular re-entry tachycardias. In this example VT (first five complexes) is converted to sinus rhythm (last three complexes) by a burst of right ventricular pacing at a rate in excess of the VT. The pacing impulses penetrate and break the re-entry circuit responsible for the VT. This permits re-establishment of sinus rhythm.

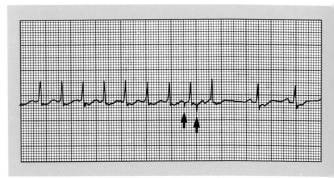

Fig.197 Premature pacing stimuli. The technique can be used for treatment of atrial or ventricular re-entry tachycardias. In this example SVT is terminated by two strategically timed atrial premature stimuli (arrowed) which penetrate and break the re-entry circuit. Sinus rhythm is thereby restored.

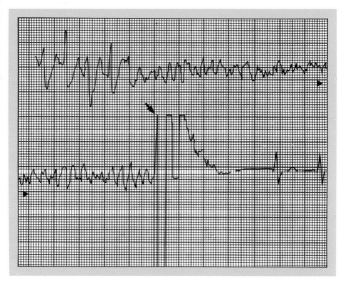

Fig.198 Direct current (DC) shock. DC depolarizes the entire myocardium and allows the sinus node to reassert itself in the majority of atrial and ventricular arrhythmias. The rapid, almost instantaneous, response to DC shock makes it treatment of choice in those tachyarrhythmias with serious haemodynamic consequences. In this example VT is seen to degenerate into VF. DC shock (arrowed) defibrillates the ventricles and after a short pause a junctional escape beat emerges re-establishing stable rhythm.

Drug treatment of atrial arrhythmias		
	Drugs	**Mechanism**
1. Prevention of arrhythmia	Disopyramide Flecainide Propafenone Amiodarone	Suppression of atrial automatic foci
2. Termination of AV nodal re-entry	Verapamil Beta-blockers	Blockade of AV conduction
3. Control of ventricular rate in atrial fibrillation	Digoxin Verapamil Beta-blockers	Blockade of AV conduction

Fig.199 Drug treatment of atrial arrhythmias. In patients with paroxysmal arrhythmias, combination therapy can be selected with the dual aim of preventing attacks and controlling the ventricular response when this fails.

Drug treatment of ventricular arrhythmias	
1. **Prevention in acute myocardial infarction**	Lignocaine Disopyramide Amiodarone
2. **Prevention in ambulant patients**	Mexiletine Disopyramide Propafenone Beta-Blockers Amiodarone
3. **Termination of established ventricular tachycardia**	Lignocaine Flecainide Amiodarone

Fig.200 Drug treatment of ventricular arrhythmias. Drugs used in ventricular arrhythmias all suppress the automaticity of ectopic foci. Great care must be taken in assessing responses to treatment since all these drugs have important proarrhythmic effects and can cause a paradoxical clinical deterioration. Proarrhythmia may be exacerbated if combination therapy is used; disopyramide and amiodarone, for example, should not be prescribed together because dangerous prolongation of the QT interval may occur, predisposing to lethal ventricular arrhythmias. Moreover, many of these drugs have negative inotropic effects, (particularly disopyramide, beta-blockers and flecainide) and must be used cautiously in heart failure.

Cardiac arrest	
Causes	Asystole Ventricular fibrillation Electromechanical dissociation
Clinical diagnosis	Absent arterial pulse Unconsciousness Apnoea
Immediate management	A. Clear airway B. Initiate ventilation (mouth-to-mouth techniques, face mask or ET tube) C. Initiate chest compression to re-establish the circulation D. Identify arrhythmia on ECG and treat appropriately

Fig.201 Cardiac arrest. Note the ABC of cardiac arrest – A airway, B breathing, and C circulation. Unskilled personnel should not waste time trying to insert an ET tube. Mouth-to-mouth techniques or a face mask are satisfactory alternatives pending the arrival of an anaesthetist. Note that ventilation and chest compression should continue uninterrupted throughout the arrest procedure.

Cardiac arrest procedures

Asystole

1. Adrenaline 1 mg – repeat every 5 minutes
2. Atropine 2 mg – if adrenaline is ineffective after 2 minutes
3. Consider DC shock (360 J) or pacing (transvenous or oesophageal)
4. Calcium chloride – only if patient is hyperkalaemic, hypocalcaemic or on calcium antagonists

Ventricular fibrillation

1. DC shock 200 J – 200 J – 360 J
2. Adrenaline 1 mg – repeat every 5 minutes
3. Repeat DC shock 360 J
4. Lignocaine 100 mg
5. Repeat DC shock 360 J
6. Consider other anti-arrhythmic drugs e.g. flecainide, amiodarone, bretyllium

Electromechanical dissociation

1. Adrenaline 1 mg IV – repeat every 5 minutes
2. Look for treatable cause – tamponade, pneumothorax, pulmonary embolism
3. Calcium chloride – only if patient is hyperkalaemic, hypocalcaemic or on calcium antagonists

Fig.202 Cardiac arrest procedures. This table summarises the main recommendations of the UK Resuscitation Council (August 1989). Note that all drugs used during a cardiac arrest should be given into a central vein. If a central line cannot be established, consider giving double doses of adrenaline, lignocaine or atropine via the endotracheal tube. In a prolonged resuscitation, IV sodium bicarbonate (50 ml of 8.3%) may be given, but ideally requirements should be titrated against blood gas analysis.

CONDUCTING TISSUE DISEASE AND PACEMAKERS

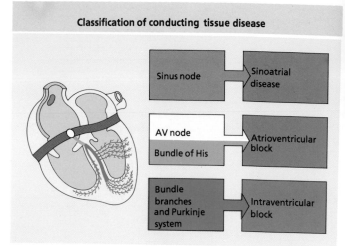

Classification of conducting tissue disease

Fig.203 Classification of conducting tissue disease. This classification provides a convenient basis for the clinical and electrocardiographic analysis of conduction defects. It must be recognized, however, that many disorders affect the conducting system at multiple levels.

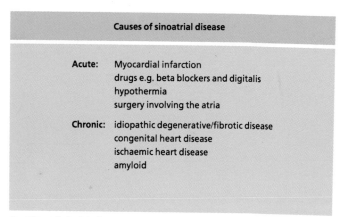

Causes of sinoatrial disease

Acute:	Myocardial infarction
	drugs e.g. beta blockers and digitalis
	hypothermia
	surgery involving the atria
Chronic:	idiopathic degenerative/fibrotic disease
	congenital heart disease
	ischaemic heart disease
	amyloid

Fig.204 Idiopathic degenerative/fibrotic disease commonly occurs in elderly patients and accounts for the majority of cases of sinoatrial dysfunction seen in clinical practice.

ECG manifestations of sinoatrial disease

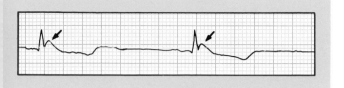

Fig.205 Sinus bradycardia – hypothermia. Since bradycardia (<50 beats/min) is physiological in athletes and healthy young people during sleep. In other circumstances it often reflects sinoatrial disease, particularly when the heart rate fails to increase normally during exercise. Here sinus bradycardia was the result of hypothermia (31°C) as evidenced by the 'J' waves at the junction of the QRS complex and the ST segment (arrowed).

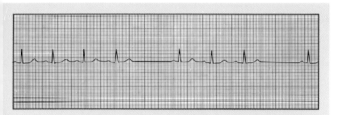

Fig.206 Sinoatrial block. In this example intermittent sinoatrial block (after the 4th and 7th complex) has prevented the sinus impulse from depolarizing the atrium. Thus no P wave is seen but because sinus discharge continues uninterrupted, the pauses are each a precise multiple of the preceeding P-P intervals. Sinoatrial block that cannot be abolished by vagal inhibition with atropine is often pathological, particularly with pauses longer than two seconds.

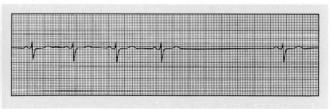

Fig.207 Sinus arrest. Failure of sinus node depolarization (sinus arrest) after the 4th complex has resulted in a pause which bears no relation to the preceeding P-P intervals. Pauses in excess of two seconds are usually pathological, particularly when they occur in the elderly. Prolonged pauses are often terminated by an escape beat from a 'junctional' (low nodal or high His bundle) focus.

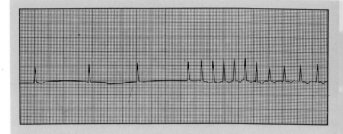

Fig.208 Bradycardia-tachycardia syndrome. In this syndrome chronic atrial (or junctional) bradycardias are interspersed with paroxysmal tachycardias. This example shows a slow junctional rhythm with the abrupt onset of rapid atrial fibrillation.

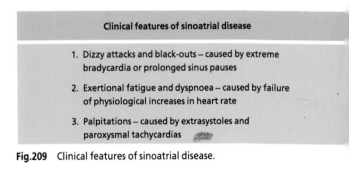

Clinical features of sinoatrial disease

1. Dizzy attacks and black-outs – caused by extreme bradycardia or prolonged sinus pauses

2. Exertional fatigue and dyspnoea – caused by failure of physiological increases in heart rate

3. Palpitations – caused by extrasystoles and paroxysmal tachycardias

Fig.209 Clinical features of sinoatrial disease.

Treatment of sinoatrial diasease

1. Pacemakers
2. Antiarrhythmic drugs
3. Anticoagulants

Fig.210 Prognosis in patients with sinoatrial disease is good (particularly in patients with idiopathic degenerative disease) and is not influenced by pacemaker therapy. Pacemaker therapy, therefore, is indicated only in symptomatic individuals to prevent dizzy attacks and blackouts and to improve exercise tolerance. Troublesome tachycardias in the bradycardia-tachycardia syndrome require antiarrhythmic drug therapy. Drugs of this type often exacerbate sinus node dysfunction and a pacemaker may be necessary to protect against severe bradycardia. Systemic emboli from the left atrium occasionally occur in the bradycardia-tachycardia syndrome and some authorities recommend prophylactic anticoagulation.

Causes of atrioventricular block	
Acute:	myocardial infarction
	drugs e.g. digitalis, verapamil
	surgery involving the high interventricular septum
Chronic:	idiopathic bilateral bundle branch fibrosis
	ischaemic heart disease
	calcific aortic and mitral valve disease
	Chagas' disease
	congenital heart disease
	connective tissue disease
	e.g. ankylosing spondylitis rheumatoid disease

Fig.211 Myocardial infarction is the commonest cause of acute AV block. Chronic AV block in this country is usually due to idiopathic disease of the bundle branches (particularly in the elderly) though ischaemic heart disease is a relatively more common cause in younger patients. Chagas' disease in S. America, however, is the commonest cause of AV block world-wide.

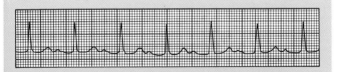

Fig.212 First degree AV block. Delayed AV conduction, as reflected by a prolonged PR interval (>0.20 secs) characterizes block of this type. The AV node is usually the site of block and ventricular depolarization occurs by normal pathways resulting in a narrow QRS complex. The condition is benign and requires no specific therapy.

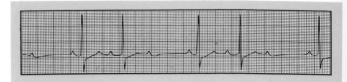

Fig.213   Second degree AV block-Mobitz type 1. Successive sinus impulses find the AV node increasingly refractory until failure of conduction occurs. The delay permits recovery of nodal function and the process may repeat itself. The ECG shows two successive cycles of Mobitz type 1 second degree AV block. Block is nearly always at nodal level and ventricular depolarization occurs by normal pathways resulting in a narrow QRS complex. The condition is common in inferior myocardial infarction, is usually transitory and requires no specific therapy.

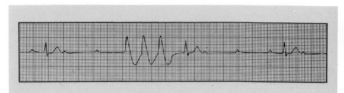

Fig.214   Second degree AV block-Mobitz type 2. Intermittent failure of AV conduction produces dropped beats. The PR interval is constant. The QRS complex may be narrow (as in this example) but is more often broad since block occurs below the junctional tissues in most cases and ventricular depolarization is by abnormal pathways. Block of this type always indicates advanced conducting tissue disease and may complicate anterior myocardial infarction. There is a significant risk of prolonged asystole. Moreover, ventricular arrhythmias occur in many cases – as illustrated by the short burst of ventricular tachycardia in this example. Pacemaker therapy is mandatory.

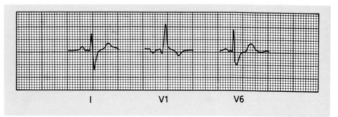

Fig.215   **Right bundle branch block (RBBB).** This may be a congenital defect but is more commonly a result of organic conducting tissue disease. Right ventricular depolarization is delayed resulting in a broad QRS complex with a large R wave in V_1, and prominent S waves in leads I and V_6. No treatment is necessary in isolated RBBB.

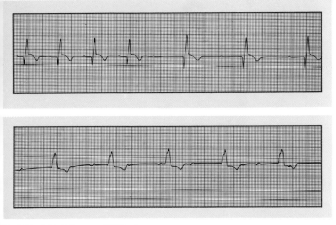

Fig.216 Third degree AV block.

a) Block at nodal level. This occurs in inferior myocardial infarction and also in most cases of congenital AV block. There is complete failure of AV conduction, but a junctional pacemaker with a reliable rate (40-70 beats/min) usually takes over. Ventricular depolarization is by normal pathways and the QRS complexes are therefore narrow. In this example the ECG (lead III) shows recent inferior myocardial infarction. The first four sinus beats are conducted with a prolonged PR interval (first degree AV block), but thereafter complete AV block develops and a slower junctional focus takes over.

b) Block at His-Purkinje level. This always indicates extensive conducting tissue disease. It may complicate anterior myocardial infarction when prognosis is poor. The ventricular escape rhythm is usually slow and unreliable with a broad QRS complex. Pacemaker therapy is mandatory.

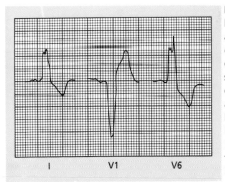

I   V1   V6

Fig.217 Left branch block (LBBB). This always indicates organic conducting tissue disease. The entire sequence of ventricular depolarization is abnormal resulting in a broad QRS complex with large slurred or notched R waves in I and V_6. No treatment is necessary in isolated LBBB.

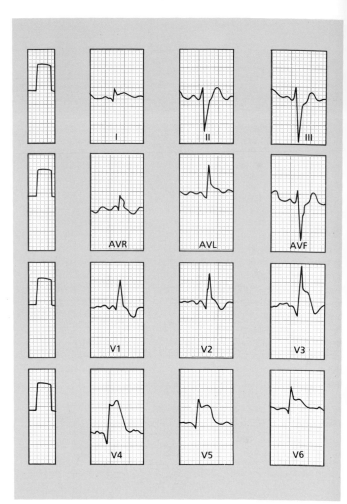

Fig.218 Bifascicular block complicating anterolateral myocardial infarction. Isolated block in either the anterior or posterior division of the left bundle is called hemiblock, and produces left or right axis deviation, respectively. When hemiblock is associated with RBBB, bifascicular block results and AV conduction is dependent on the remaining division of the left bundle. The danger of complete AV block developing in this situation is considerable, particularly if bifascicular block is a complication of acute myocardial infarction when prophylactic pacemaker therapy is indicated. In other contexts no treatment is necessary unless progression to complete AV block occurs.

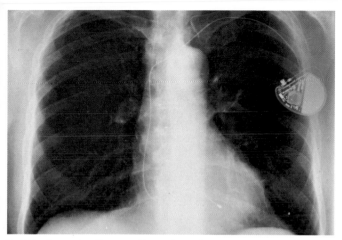

Fig.219 Pacemaker therapy – the equipment.
Permanent pacing. The chest radiograph shows a permanent pacemaker system. The power source (or generator) is situated subcutaneously below the left clavicle and attached to a lead with a terminal electrode positioned in the apex of the right ventricle. The generator delivers electric pulses which depolarize the ventricles.
Temporary pacing. Temporary pacing is used when the need for rate control is likely to be only transient (e.g. heart block in inferior infarction) or as a prelude to permanent pacing in patients with severe bradycardias. An external power source is used. This is attached to a transvenous wire positioned in the right ventricle.

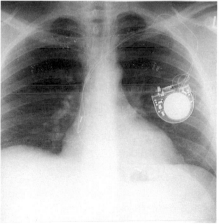

Fig.220 Physiological (DDD) pacing. The pacemaker generator is in the left pectoral position and is attached to two wires positioned in the right atrium and right ventricle. Systems of this type re-establish normal atrial and ventricular synchrony in complete AV block and are being used increasingly, particularly in younger patients.

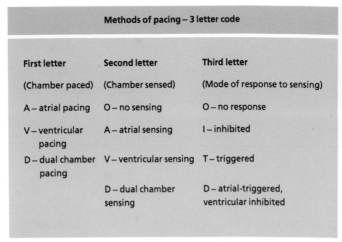

Methods of pacing – 3 letter code		
First letter	**Second letter**	**Third letter**
(Chamber paced)	(Chamber sensed)	(Mode of response to sensing)
A – atrial pacing	O – no sensing	O – no response
V – ventricular pacing	A – atrial sensing	I – inhibited
D – dual chamber pacing	V – ventricular sensing	T – triggered
	D – dual chamber sensing	D – atrial-triggered, ventricular inhibited

Fig.221 Methods of pacing – 3 letter code. Fixed rate ventricular pacing (VOO) is now never used and the majority of modern units are either VVI or DDD (see below).

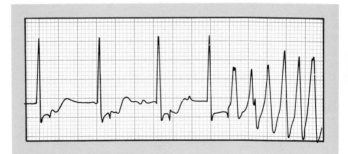

Fig.222 Fixed rate ventricular pacing (VOO). The potential dangers of VOO pacing are illustrated here. The fixed rate pacing artefact is seen early after each QRS complex when the ventricle is refractory and unresponsive. However, electrical stimulation in this 'vulnerable period' of the cardiac cycle is dangerous and eventually triggers rapid ventricular tachycadia.

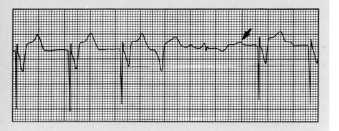

Fig.223 Ventricular inhibited demand pacing (VVI). The first three complexes are paced: the complexes are broad, confirming their ventricular origin, and each is preceded by a pacing artefact. A spontaneous ventricular premature beat then inhibits the pacemaker and is followed by a sinus beat conducted with delay (prolonged PR interval). The next sinus impulse is not conducted and the ventricular pacemaker takes over again. Note that in VVI pacing, spontaneous ventricular beats inhibit the pacemaker, ensuring that pacing impulses do not fall during the vulnerable period of the cardiac cycle.

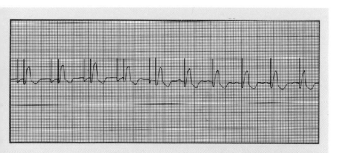

Fig.224 Dual demand pacing (DDD). Conventional ventricular pacing with a VVI unit does not restore synchronous atrial contraction in AV block. DDD pacing, however, re-establishes the normal atrioventricular relationship by delivering impulses with physiological delay, first to the right atrium and then to the ventricle ('sequential pacing'). Alternatively, if normal atrial activity is intact 'synchronized' pacing may be used which senses atrial depolarization and then stimulates the ventricle, again with appropriate delay. Clearly DDD pacing cannot be used in patients with atrial fibrillation. In the illustration the first five complexes are each preceded by two pacing artefacts, indicating sequential AV pacing. Thereafter the intrinsic sinus rate accelerates and the pre-programmed pacemaker changes to synchronized node sensing the P wave and pacing the ventricle.

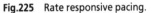

Rate responsive pacing	
Responses to exertion which trigger rate increase	**Pacing method**
1. Increasing atrial rate	DDD
2. Shortening QT interval	VVI
3. Somatic vibrations	VVI
4. Falling venous pH	Not commercially available
5. Rising body temperature	Not commercially available

Fig.225 Rate responsive pacing.

Pacemakers are now available which sense a physiological response to exertion and respond with a graded increase in rate. DDD pacemakers are rate responsive because as the atrial rate increases so the rate of the triggered ventricular response increases. However, these pacemakers depend upon dual atrial and ventricular electrodes and an intact atrial rhythm. More recently rate-responsive VVI pacemakers have become available, sensing either exertional alterations in the QT interval or somatic vibrations and responding with an increase in rate. Rate-responsive pacing improves exercise tolerance and is recommended in young active patients.

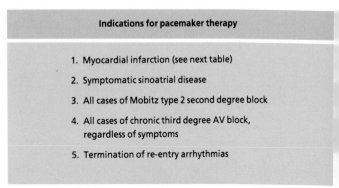

Indications for pacemaker therapy
1. Myocardial infarction (see next table)
2. Symptomatic sinoatrial disease
3. All cases of Mobitz type 2 second degree block
4. All cases of chronic third degree AV block, regardless of symptoms
5. Termination of re-entry arrhythmias

Fig.226 Indications for pacemaker therapy.

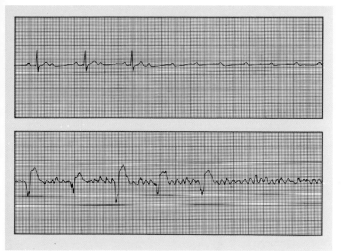

Fig.227 These ECGs provide graphic illustration of the importance of pacemaker therapy in Mobitz type 2 and complete AV block. In the first example, Mobitz type 2 block gives way to complete failure of AV conduction with prolonged asystole. In the second example, the atrium is fibrillating but complete AV block is evident by the *regular* broad complex ventricular rhythm. Again the rhythm strip terminates with prolonged asystole. In both cases a pacemaker would have been life saving.

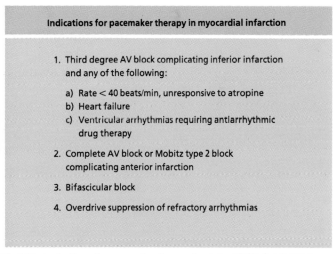

Indications for pacemaker therapy in myocardial infarction

1. Third degree AV block complicating inferior infarction and any of the following:

   a) Rate < 40 beats/min, unresponsive to atropine
   b) Heart failure
   c) Ventricular arrhythmias requiring antiarrhythmic drug therapy

2. Complete AV block or Mobitz type 2 block complicating anterior infarction

3. Bifascicular block

4. Overdrive suppression of refractory arrhythmias

Fig.228 Indications for pacemaker therapy in myocardial infarction.

MISCELLANEOUS CARDIAC DISORDERS

Adult congenital heart disease

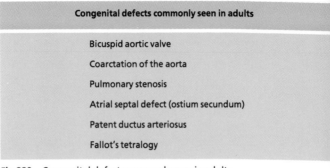

Congenital defects commonly seen in adults
Bicuspid aortic valve
Coarctation of the aorta
Pulmonary stenosis
Atrial septal defect (ostium secundum)
Patent ductus arteriosus
Fallot's tetralogy

Fig.229 Congenital defects commonly seen in adults.

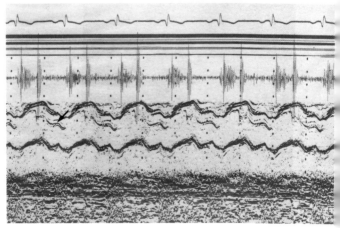

Fig.230 Bicuspid aortic valve. In this M-mode echocardiogram in an asymptomatic young adult the diastolic closure line of the aortic valve (arrowed) lies eccentrically within the aortic root suggesting a bicuspid valve. The valve is normal in other respects. The ejection click and murmur typical of this condition are recorded on the phonocardiogram. Turbulent flow across the bicuspid valve progressively traumatizes the leaflets which fibrose and calcify leading to stenosis in middle-age.

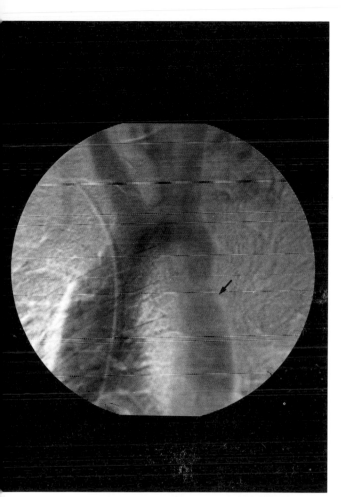

Fig.231 Coarctation of the aorta – aortogram. This digital subtraction study in a young man shows a discrete coarctation (arrowed) in the thoracic aorta. Flow into the abdominal aorta is restricted and the femoral pulse is delayed and diminished. Renal hypoperfusion activitates the renin-angiotensin system and leads to hypertension. Deaths from LVF or cerebral haemorrhage usually occurs in middle-age unless surgical correction is undertaken. Coarctation is often associated with other congenital defects. In this example there was a bicuspid aortic valve (the commonest associated abnormality) which was significantly stenosed. Post-stenotic dilatation of the ascending aorta is clearly seen.

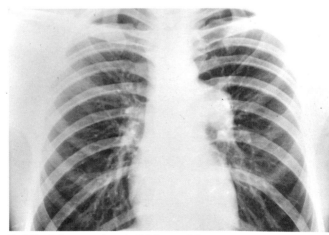

Fig.232 Coarctation: aortogram. Contrast has been injected through a catheter advanced into the thoracic aorta from the femoral artery. In this case the thoracic aorta was completely occluded by the coarctation. Note the large collaterals bypassing the coarctation and feeding into the distal aorta. These are responsible for the rib-notching commonly seen on the chest X-ray.

Fig.233 Pulmonary stenosis. This is one of the more common congenital defects seen in adults. The chest X-ray shows post-stenotic dilatation of the pulmonary artery. In most cases no treatment is necessary but in severe pulmonary stenosis surgical correction is required. Balloon valvuloplasty has largely replaced surgery for the treatment of pulmonary stenosis in infants.

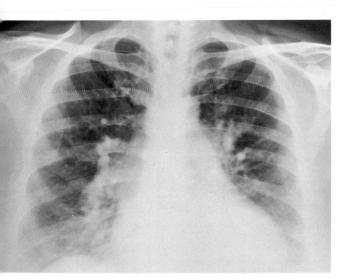

Fig.234 Atrial septal defect – chest X-ray. Note the prominent proximal pulmonary arteries and the pulmonary plethora reflecting increased pulmonary flow.

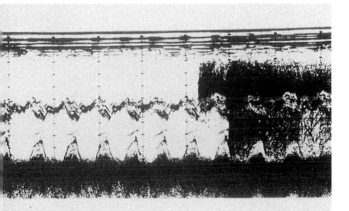

Fig.235 Atrial septal defect: contrast echocardiogram. Hand-agitated saline solution has been injected into a peripheral vein. Bubble contrast appears first in the right side of the heart (anteriorly) and shortly afterwards in the left side (posteriorly) due to shunting of bubbles across an atrial septal defect. Note how the volume-loaded right ventricle is dilated compared with the left ventricle.

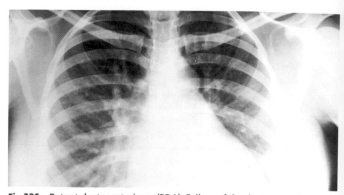

Fig.236 Patent ductus arteriosus (PDA). Failure of the ductus arteriosus closure in the neonate results in a left to right shunt between the aorta and the pulmonary artery. If the shunt is large, heart failure and pulmonary vascular disease develop. Chest X-ray in this adult woman shows a thin line of calcification just below the aortic knuckle. This is the 'comma' sign and represents a calcified PDA. Cardiomegaly and pulmonary plethora indicate that the shunt is large. Surgical correction is necessary regardless of the size of the shunt, because of the risk of endocarditis.

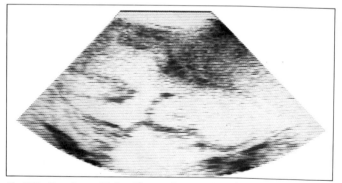

Fig.237 Tetralogy of Fallot. The tetralogy consists of ventricular septal defect, pulmonary stenosis, dilatation and dextraposition of the aorta (which overrides the septal defect) and right ventricular hypertrophy. Pulmonary stenosis is usually severe and increases RV pressure sufficiently to produce right to left shunting across the VSD. This results in cyanosis. In less severe cases the shunt is from left to right (acyanotic Fallot's). The 2D echocardiogram (long-axis view) shows the VSD and the dilated aorta overriding the defect. Complete surgical correction of Fallot's tetralogy is now possible and should be undertaken in all cases.

Aortic dissection

Clinical presentation of aortic dissection
1. Chest pain
2. Regional arterial insufficiency
3. Aortic regurgitation
4. Cardiac tamponade
5. Sudden death

Fig.238 In patients with degenerative disease of the aortic media, an intimal tear allows high pressure arterial blood to create a false lumen for a variable distance through the aortic media. The tear is usually proximal, just above the aortic valve, but may be more distal particularly in hypertensive patients. Partial or complete occlusion of branch arteries arising from the aorta leads to regional ischaemia while disruption of the aortic valve ring produces aortic regurgitation. External rupture into the pericardial or pleural spaces is common and often fatal. Where possible, surgical repair should be undertaken, particularly in proximal dissections.

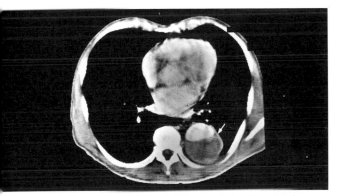

Fig.239 Aortic dissection – CAT scan. In this example the dissection has extended into the descending thoracic aorta (arrowed) which is considerably dilated. Contrast enhancement clearly separates the true and false lumens.

Pulmonary thromboembolism

Clinical presentation of pulmonary thromboembolism

Symptoms   Chest pain*

Dyspnoea*
Cough*
Haemoptysis
Syncope

Signs   Tachypnoea*
Loud S2 (pulmonary component)*
Tachycardia
JVP
Gallop rhythm
Signs of DVT
Cyanosis

* present in > 50% of patients with pulmonary embolism

Fig.240   Clinical presentation. Pulmonary thromboembolism usually derives from the deep veins of the legs or pelvis. It is a common cause of hospital morbidity and mortality. The severity of the clinical presentation relates to the extent of pulmonary vascular obstruction but the symptoms and signs are very variable and usually nondiagnostic.

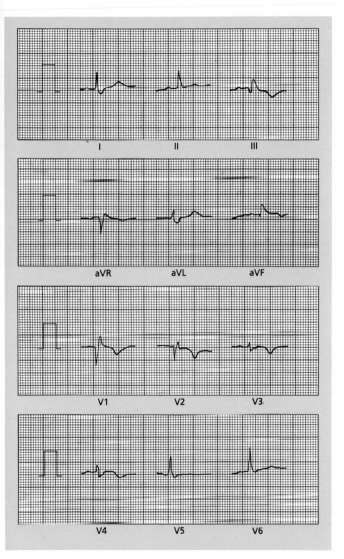

Fig.241 ECG. The ECG changes in pulmonary embolism are as variable as the clinical findings and are nondiagnostic. Classically, however, the changes reflect RV strain as illustrated in this example from a patient with massive pulmonary embolism. Note the S1, Q3, T3 pattern with incomplete RBBB. T wave inversion in V1 to V4 is a further manifestation of RV strain.

ANTERIOR

Perfusion　　　　　　　　　　　　　Ventilation

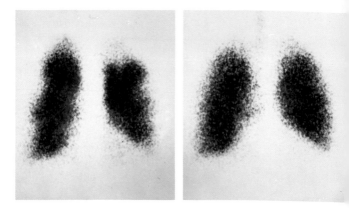

POSTERIOR

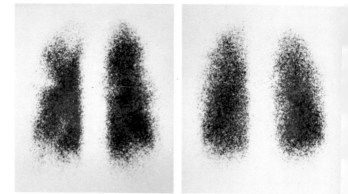

Fig.242　Ventilation-perfusion isotope lung scan. In pulmonary embolism, alveolar ventilation remains normal and the ventilation scan shows homogeneous distribution of isotope. Blood flow to those parts of the lung subtended by the obstructed vessel (or vessels), however, is impaired and the perfusion scan shows regional defects. The demonstration of ventilation-perfusion 'mismatch' is highly specific for pulmonary embolism. In this example ventilation scans are on the right and perfusion scans are on the left. Several areas of mismatch are seen indicating multiple pulmonary emboli.

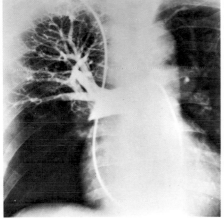

Fig.243 Pulmonary angiogram. There is complete obstruction of the left pulmonary artery and also of the branches to the right, middle and lower lobes. Only the right upper lobe branches are patent. The patient had suffered massive pulmonary embolism and later died.

Cardiac tumours

Classification of primary cardiac tumours	
Benign	Myxoma
	Lipoma
	Rhabdomyoma
	Fibroma
Malignant	Angiosarcoma
	Rhabdomyosarcoma
	Fibrosarcoma

Fig.244 Malignant disease of the heart is usually due to secondary invasion, often from the breast or lung. Primary cardiac tumours are rare, the most common being the histologically benign myxoma.

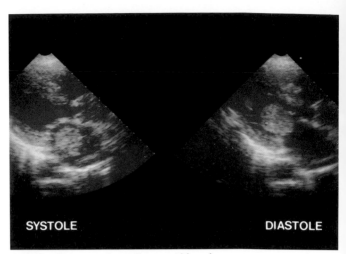

Fig.245 Myxoma – echocardiogram. Although myxomas may occur in any of the cardiac chambers, the majority are left atrial and present with symptoms and signs that are almost indistinguishable from mitral stenosis. These 2D echocardiograms in systole and diastole show a left atrial myxoma. Note that during diastole the tumour prolapses through the mitral valve obstructing LV filling as if the valve were stenosed.

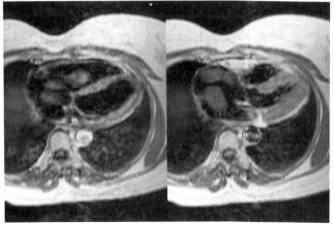

Fig.246 Left atrial myxoma – magnetic resonance imaging. This is a new technique providing high resolution cardiac images. In this example a lobulated myxoma is clearly seen within the left atrium. During diastole (left frame) one lobe prolapses through the mitral valve.

INDEX